The
Minimalism
Effect

Brett Turley

ISBN: 1502712555
ISBN-13: 978-1502712554

DEDICATION

The Minimalism Effect is dedicated to my father, Phil. Without his minimalistic attitude towards living and his constant voice in my head to push and be better I would not have accomplished what I have done today let alone put this book together. You may not be here anymore, but you are always with me.

The Minimalism Effect

Brett Turley

CONTENTS

Brett Turley

ACKNOWLEDGMENTS

Firstly acknowledgement must go to those who are smarter, more accomplished and capable than myself. This began from an idea at my father's kitchen table after my second tour of Afghanistan but was inspired and invigorated by the works and teaching of people mentioned within this book. Going against the status quo of the fitness industry was the path less traveled but it has made all the difference.

Photos for the cover of The Minimalism Effect are by Anna Brown from Black Box Photography. *Thanks Anna.*

Lastly, to my wife Jo, thanks for putting up with the countless days of sitting in the office swearing at the computer.

Minimalism –

"A design or style where the simplest and fewest elements are used to create the maximum effect." – Websters Dictionary

Brett Turley

1 THE PHILOSPHY

Less is More.

1. Begin with the end in mind.
2. Put first things first.
3. Be like water; adjust accordingly to achieve what you set out to do.
4. Add nothing that is unnecessary to achieve your goals.
5. Stay the course and finish what you have started.

Inside this book you will find useful information to help you achieve your fitness goals. Some of which you will like and some of which you won't pay any attention to at all. Take what you want from the text, programs and demonstrations and if you find a better way, use it.

The idea is simple; reduce the amount of elements in your training program that dilutes the outcome. Focus on the few, small but important elements and do them well. Take time to invest in your learning to master these skills and you will be better. You can start where you wish throughout the book. The main concern is that once you have started a program you must commit to mastering it. This will be a paradigm shift for most due to the constant state of flux within people's lives and their inability to see things through. Challenge yourself to master everything in this book and you will be better by doing less.

To master the principle of minimalism you must master patience, perseverance and competence. It will be a long road but master a few essential skills as opposed to dabbling in a lot of things will serve you well for application in not only fitness training but life in general.

How I became a Minimalist

It's a story of pain and sorrow…. Not really, I just got tired of getting injured. My wrap sheet is long and distinguished in the injury department:

- 13 shoulder dislocations,
- 1 shoulder reconstruction,
- Dislocated and fractured ankle,
- Numerous sprains, strains both chronic and acute,
- And the list goes on.

This all came from a balls-to-the-wall lifestyle and training regime. Joining the Army at age 17 did not help when I had people in my ear telling me to "Go harder for longer you pussy."

This probably stemmed from earlier years of competitive rugby and keeping up with blokes twice my size. This takes its toll on the body but I had finally had enough on my second tour of Afghanistan. In chronic pain from my sciatic nerve walking 20km with 30-40kg of gear on my back and having my trusty explosive detection dog "Bullseye" off my hip and in 40-degree heat I thought to myself there must be a better way. Sporting a sweet set of orthotics I was recommended to wear by some Army doctor, training to my limit every session between jobs out of the wire, the pain just wouldn't go away. And then it hit me.

"Less is More."

I got rid of the orthotics, bought a pair of minimalist shoes and sooner rather than later I was pain free. From then on I started to educate myself with training strategies that promote recovery and longevity as opposed to squeezing every last rep out of the day. I haven't looked back, pain free for the majority of the time as there have been some speed bumps but hey, that's learning for you. I am now the strongest, fastest and most mobile I have ever been. Although old habits die hard, which I know yours will too. I eventually saw that this was the path for me, just like all of my clients and their amazing success stories.

So you too can rid your body of injury and become the strongest and most able you have ever been by using this philosophy. It has worked for hundreds, if not thousands before you.

Brett Turley

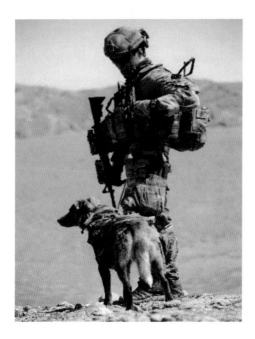

Afghanistan 2012 – Explosive Detection Dog "Bullseye". I trained and deployed with this little guy, one of the most loyal companions I have ever known.

Bodyweight, Kettlebells & Barbell Training – Is that all?

The simplest and fewest elements used to create the maximum effect. That is the sole focus of the whole program. Instead of adding ridiculous amounts of clutter within your training program, making you focus on the few essential elements and skills will ensure progression and success over your training period.

Too many people these days search for the quick fix or the latest technology to help them get to where they want to be, by removing these temptations and by outlining a simple yet effective program you will be able to see that all of these "gadgets" for "fads" are no longer needed. The idea is to simplify ones life and be master of the basics.

But do not be deceived some of these basics have been around for hundreds of years and guess what the reason is?

Because they work.

Points to remember

1. It all begins with movement. Ever since childhood we have based everything on movement. Before we add strength or performance to an exercise or skill we must first master being able to move competently. Missing this first and most crucial element will lead to only two outcomes:

- Injury and or;
- Poor Performance.

Do not be hasty when it comes to movement. From the mouth of Gray Cook, "move well and then move often". This embodies the three key stages to mastering minimalism, patience, perseverance and competence. If you follow this path all the strength and performance you desire will follow and probably more.

2. General Physical Preparedness (GPP) vs. Specific Physical Preparedness (SPP) – Elite athletes this isn't you. Although an athlete would get a lot out of this in terms of injury prevention and progressions and regressions for their training cycles this wasn't designed for someone performing at an elite level. As it was *phrased* on my Russian Kettlebell Certification (RKC) by Andrew Read:

"So what makes you an elite athlete? You get paid for what you do, and you don't need a second job to get your bills paid."

The Minimalism Effect is targeting GPP. It is designed for the beginner to intermediate athlete or individual that wants to be good at a range of qualities and be able to adapt to anything. Someone who is at the very beginning of their career, either a teenager or youth athlete or an adult that is looking to make his or her body an adaptable, durable and injury free machine.

If you are an elite athlete, take what you want from this book and leave the rest. You should be targeting SPP. To be truly great you only need to focus your efforts on what will have direct results on your performance. Chances are your coach will tell you this anyway, if not, fire your coach!

3. Don't overdraw your bank account. However you need to condition your mind, internalize the attitude that fitness is for tomorrow, not today. If you go maxing out everyday in training you won't leave anything in the tank for game day or testing.

"Fitness is meant to fill the tank, always leave reps or in the bank saving them for when you need them most. So you don't run out of fuel on game day."

All good coaches will say the same thing, so they must be onto something. I need to reiterate this point because I want it to set in:

Fitness is a bank account. You need to make regular deposits so it increases in equity. The more you draw against that equity the less you will have and before you know it, you will be overdrawn. This means an injury or burn out.

4. Don't re-invent the wheel. All this stuff has been around for decades and the reason it is still around is because it works. Time tested and proven strategies that have had far smarter and more capable men prove them right time and time again. A lot of this stuff in this book has helped me achieve all the standards within this book and my clients have achieved many of the same. If you wish to further your knowledge into a particular field,

educate yourself with whoever sparks your interest. There is a list of further reading at the back of the book.

5. Get a god damn coach. At any point if you feel you haven't or aren't hitting the mark with your training, get a coach. They will accelerate your progress and pick up things you would never have thought about. A good coach will not let you make the same mistakes as they did. Look for someone that specializes in what you need help with.

A good coach will be able to deliver cues and tips either verbally, visually or kinesthetically that will prompt the desired results or effect.

You will notice in the book that some of the techniques for the programs are not there; there is a reason for this. Many people only absorb 20% of what is written in text within a book. This highlights the need to get a coach and learn correctly the first time. You can employ the services of anyone who is qualified in these areas. Think of it as an investment into injury prevention and future greatness. Learning things correctly the first time will save you a lot of money down the track and will help you avoid injury.

6. Stay the course. Start to finish, surrender to the process and enjoy the adventure and it will be worth it.

2 THE STANDARDS & SKILLS

The Standards

Standards are essential. They let you know where you sit in the world and where your short falls lie. These standards are adapted from Dan John's *Intervention*, the women's section is allocated by me and have held true for many of my own clients:

First of note is a score of 14 or above on the Functional Movement Screen (FMS) with no asymmetries. For both male and female.

For Men –

Push – Bodyweight Bench Press

Advanced – Bodyweight (BW) Bench Press 15 Repetitions

Pull – 8-10 Pull-ups

Advanced – 15 Pull-ups

Squat – Bodyweight Squat (SQ)

Advanced – BW SQ 15 Reps

Hip Hinge – 150% Bodyweight Deadlift (DL)

Advanced – 200% BW DL

Loaded Carry – 30m Bodyweight Farmers Walk (split across both hands)

Advanced – 30m 200% BW Farmers Walk

For Women –

Push – 75% BW Bench Press

Advanced – BW Bench Press

Pull – 1 Pull-up

Advanced – 3 Pull-ups

Squat – 50% BW Squat 5 Reps

Advanced – BW SQ

Hip Hinge – Bodyweight DL

Advanced – 150% BW DL

Loaded Carry – 30m Farmers Walk BW

Advanced – 30m BW and a half Farmers Walk

You should attempt to make these standards. If you achieve the advanced standards you will be in a rare class, which is regarded as strong enough for anything. Additionally standards you should aim for using the Minimalism Effect are:

Brett Turley

For Men –

Half Bodyweight Kettlebell Press

Half Bodyweight Get Up

For Women –

24kg Kettlebell Press

24kg Get Up

Additional –

One Arm Push-up

One Arm Pull-up

Pistol Squat

Hanging Leg Raise

Bridge

Handstand Push-ups

If you manage to achieve all of the strength feats above you will be stronger than almost 99% of the worlds population. You will be able to dazzle your friends with your skills and be able to adapt to almost any sport with relative ease. The emphasis should be placed on skill and technique, take your time to master at least the basic strength standards and you will be rewarded for it.

The Skills

Along this journey we always place the emphasis on skill and technique. Mastering movement and technique always trumps, muscling through a movement. Strength will progress far quicker when you pay attention to the finer details. Below is a table I use to screen clients when they first come in for training, it gives me a snap shot of what they know, where we need to start and where their short falls lie. Almost universally, everyone starts from scratch.

Squat	Hip Hinge	Push
Toe Touch	Hip Hinge Patterning	Push-up Plank
Goblet Squat	Romanian Deadlift	Push-up
Face the Wall Squat	KB Suitcase Deadlift	KB Floor Press
Single KB Rack Squat	Single Leg Deadlift	Bench Press
DBL KB Rack Squat	Barbell Deadlift	DBL KB Press
Front Squat	KB Swing	Bottoms Up Press
Back Squat	KB Clean	Single KB Press
Overhead Squat	KB Snatch	Barbell Press

Pull	Loaded Carry	Everything Else
KB Bat Wing Row	Farmers Walk	Crocodile Breathing
Inverted Row	Rack Walk	Soft Rolling
Renegade Row	Overhead Walk	Hard Rolling
Active Hang	Prowler Push	Rocking
Static Hold	Sled Pull/Walk	Bear Crawl
Jack Knife Pull-ups	Suitcase Walk	Lateral Swing/Hang
Chin-ups	Rack Walk	Hanging Leg Raise
Pull-ups	Single KB Waiter Walk	Get Up
Weighted Pull-ups	Hill Sprints	Windmill

There are some progressions of our exercises that you will not need to master during your training straight away. Things like the overhead squat lead into our explosive or Olympic style lifts and require a lot of skill and movement competency, these are for another book within itself. Ask yourself the question; are these absolutely necessary to achieving the requirements in the strength standards?

If not, don't bother. Spend your time on the movements and exercises that target your specific goals. Tick them off when you complete them. You may need to advance some skills quicker than others in your training, which is allowed. Note that these are skills and not lifts you must be attaining personal records in, the idea is to master each skill set and then set your personal records. This may happen at the start or end of your training.

3 GETTING STARTED

You are already equipped with the equipment you need to start, your body. Start wherever you choose throughout the book but if cash is tight, start on the Evolution of Man. As you progress and master the program you can then consider purchasing your first pieces of equipment or a gym membership. Here is a list of the first pieces of equipment you should start with:

- Foam Roller
- Massage Ball
- Kettlebells – Women 8kg, 12kg & 16kg/Men 16kg, 20kg & 24kg
- Gymnastics Rings
- Skipping rope
- Powerbands
- Dowel

You will see what the equipment will be used for in later chapters. For the barbell section if you don't want to spend too much money on expensive equipment then a cheap membership to a 24hr fitness club will do the trick, this is probably the only time that I would ever recommend using one. You can also purchase double kettlebells for your chosen weight if you feel inclined to do so, but you can achieve most goals with a single bell.

Brett Turley

I would personally recommend starting on the prehabilitation program, take the time to bulletproof your body for the upcoming training. This will also get a start on the basics of kettlebells, saving you time down the road. Don't forget if you need a coach get one.

The Phases

The following is a suggested breakdown of where to put each program. Some may take longer to achieve certain goals and some may get through quicker. You can also start where you want. The lay out is dominated by progression of skills and longevity in training but some skills will require a quicker advance than others.

Phase One: Prehab Program

Phase Two: Evolution of Man

Phase Three: Kettlebell Fundamentals

Phase Four: 6-week Minimalist Barbell Cycle

Phase Five: Barbell Cycle with Alternate Big Three

Phase Six: Minimalistic Rite Of Passage

Phase Seven: Kettlebell Hell

Phases six and seven can be switched depending on your preference. Following this sequence will give you a minimum of 10-11 months of training. Anyone who knows about the ups and downs of life will know that this will equate to a full year at least. Realistically if you could achieve all the standards in 18 months you are doing well.

4 BULLETPROOFING

In this phase you will find all you need to know to start forging a body that can take all sorts of punishment. It will contain warm-up strategies, correctives to help you fix asymmetries and imbalances within your body and exercises to make you a better, well-rounded athlete. Remember when it comes to correctives; do not add excessive load to the activity and good correctives can also be exercises in the body of a session.

Best Correctives Are Warm Ups

Your best time to use correctives is during your warm-up. After foam rolling, mobility work and myofascial compression techniques (MCT) your body will be ready to start absorbing what you are trying to teach or correct. It is important to focus on correctives that will have an effect on your individual issues and prepare you for the session ahead. To start off on the right foot you may need to do something first.

Get An FMS

Getting a Functional Movement Screen or FMS before you begin a phase of your training is a great way to get a snapshot of how well you are moving and to see if there are any asymmetries or limitations within certain movement patterns or areas of the body. Using this screen to help decide what corrective strategy is appropriate will help you and save you mountains of wasted time when it comes to structuring the correct warm-up. You can find FMS certified coaches in most cities visit functionalmovement.com to find an FMS certified instructor near you.

Brett Turley

Structure Of A Warm Up

The structure of a warm-up is just as important as the structure of the body of a session. It helps you work on your weaker areas and prepares you adequately for later work. Cutting short your warm-up is not advised as many people before you have seen the consequences of a poorly structured or inadequate warm-up. Just go visit your local physiotherapist for further case studies. So here is the structure of a warm up:

1.   **Joint Assessment** – involves taking your joints through their Range of Motion (ROM) and to identify any potential issues that may affect your training. I usually move from bottom to top to help clients remember the sequence. Ankles, knees, hips, shoulders, elbows, wrists and neck. There are many ways you can do this; many of your correctives will also help you identify any issues with your joints.
2.   **Foam Roll/MCT** – foam rolling or trigger point therapy on areas that are tight or need working out. Muscle adhesions or 'knots' as many people like to call them will form in areas that have an existing injury, that are tight from subsequent sessions or from areas that have been neglected previously. Take the time to hit all the areas of concern. There are heaps of tools you can use for this such as foam rollers, stick rollers and trigger point balls.
3.   **Corrective Work** – This is where we place the bulk of our focus. When conducted correctly most corrective work will be an adequate warm up for most activity. We will address mobility and motor control issues within our movement patterns, focusing on areas highlighted by our FMS. We may use a variety of techniques for corrective work such as Proprioceptive Neuromuscular Facilitation (PNF) and Reactive Neuromuscular Training (RNT). The important thing is we address mobility issues first followed by motor control. For further information on this get in touch with an FMS certified instructor or better yet, take the course yourself. The knowledge gained from a course like this is invaluable.
4.   **General Warm-Up** – If you feel that your corrective work has not quite hit the mark, you can use things like the rower or skipping to get you moving, the simple premise for this section is get your heart rate up but do not add excessive load.
5.   **Specific Warm-Up** – Here we target direct competencies required for our given session. If we are using kettlebells this can include but is not

limited to hip hinge patterning or goblet squats. This will also include dynamic movements if you are sprinting or training power based movements. This can include your preparation sets for lifting.

Foam Rolling, Mobilization & Static Stretching For Cool Downs

Weird place to put it but your cool down can sometimes mirror parts of your warm-up as an active recovery to spin down from exercise. There has been numerous studies into the effectiveness of static stretching in both warm-ups and cool downs. I believe they should be applied during your cool down and once educated correctly you can apply some to your warm-up. For now, stick to the warm-up breakdown given and add some foam rolling, mobilization and static stretching in your cool down. Hitting the pool for a cool down isn't a bad idea either or even just for a recovery session. If you live near the beach or a pool, hit the water after a session to help those muscles recover.

Sub Your Rest For Correctives

When you are training with large amounts of rest periods don't be afraid to add a few correctives. Target the movement or skills you are using with your corrective strategy. This will help improve your performance during your training and help get more corrective work into your routine. You can never move well enough.

The Correctives and Exercises

The following pages you will find mountains of interesting exercises that will help you move better. Take the time to explore them and find the ones that seem to help you the most. Having a functional movement screen conducted by an FMS certified instructor would show you what you have to focus on and address.

The correctives and drills featured will address different issues certain areas of the body or movement patterns. The first section will address predominantly mobility and motor control issues within sections of the body; the second will address core/midsection static and dynamic motor control issues to link both top and bottom. The reason this section is important is because of the philosophy of training muscles and not movement patterns, your body quite often becomes disconnected from its upper and lower. This will help correct these issues of imbalances and asymmetries. The final section is based on movement patterns and will link the previous mobility and core/midsection areas together into functional patterns and once again correcting mobility and motor control issues promoting correct technique.

Breathing

Breathing is the basis of all movement. Without the ability to breathe correctly you can cause numerous issues such as restricted range of motion to early fatigue during exercise. The crocodile breathing drill will help develop diaphragmatic breathing to enhance your movement and performance by utilizing a full breathing pattern as opposed to being restricted during breathing.

Crocodile Breathing

• Lay face down or prone on the floor with your forehead on your hands.

• Using the floor as a way of gaining proprioceptive feedback or more feeling, breathe in through your nose and fill your stomach.

• Your stomach should push into the floor making your abdominal cavity tighter. Avoid initiating the breath with your mouth or rising at the chest.

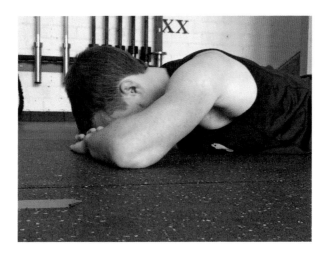

•   From here imagine a crocodile lying on the bank, you should start to breath into your flanks or sides, the part to aim to fill is the gap between ribs and hips.

•   Your stomach should feel like it is getting tighter, abdominal bracing from this type of breathing will give you the feeling that your mid section is bound together and tight.

Once you have developed this laying on your stomach technique, attempt to breath like this while standing or in various other positions such as supine (laying on your back), quadruped, kneeling or standing. Diaphragmatic breathing will help you maintain abdominal bracing throughout movement and exercise. Efforts should be made at all times to keep this breathing pattern. The use of diaphragmatic breathing or power breaths in high tension exercises such as kettlebell ballistics and maximal type lifts is essential for safe and strong lifting.

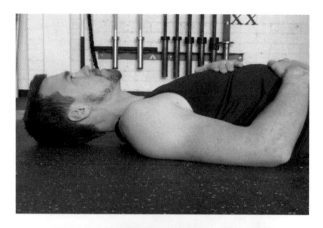

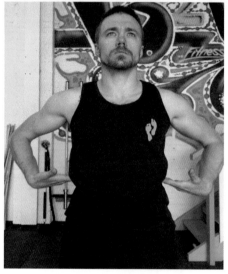

Figure 1: demonstrates Crocodile breathing in a supine position and Figure 2: demonstrates in a standing position using the hands to feel the correct breathing sequence.

Hips & Posterior Chain

When dealing with poor flexibility or mobility it doesn't always come from the area detected as tight or sore. Referral pain, pain that is transmitted to another area by a separate cause often misleads people into thinking they have problems when the problem is in a completely different area. A sore or tight lower back is one of the most common complaints and problems with clients. People that work in sedentary jobs or spend all day in an office at a desk tend to neglect the hips by being in a slouched over position in a chair or desk. The following exercises are for people to address complaints such as these and this is why the hips and posterior chain have been put in the same category.

Leg Lowering

• Using a resistance band, loop the band around and over your foot, holding onto it with both hands.

• Leaving both knees locked and feet pulled back towards the body or in dorsiflexion, raise the leg with the band to a comfortable height where the knee does not bend but a stretch can be felt.

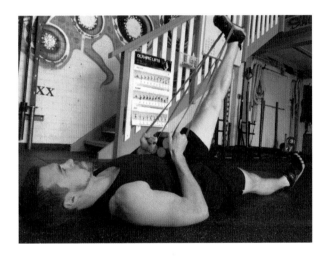

• From here, raise the opposite leg meeting the height of the banded leg without the knees bending. Return to the floor with the moving leg without letting the foot slap against the floor.

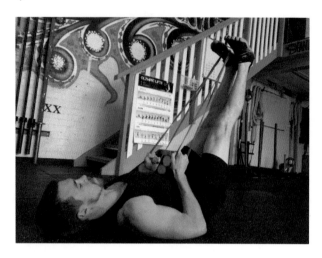

•   Efforts should be made to keep the toes flexed back towards the body at all times.

•   As you feel the muscles lengthen increase the height at which you hold the banded leg.

•   Complete enough repetitions that an increase in mobility can be noticed, usually 10-20 repetitions each leg.

•   You can also do this in a doorway or without the banded leg support.

ASLR with Core Activation

ASLR stands for Active Straight Leg Raise.

•   For this corrective you will require two resistance bands of equal size. Mount them on a vertical structure at approximately hip height.

•   Lie in a supine position far enough away to have the arms in a vertical position with a small amount of resistance on the bands.

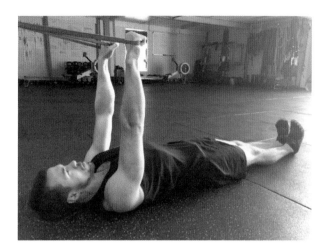

• Once in the correct position you are to breath into your mid section and brace, you then bring both arms down to the side of the body locking them into place.

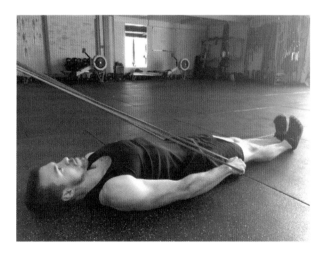

• Next, use a leg raise in similar fashion to the leg lowering drill, bringing one leg up as high as you can.

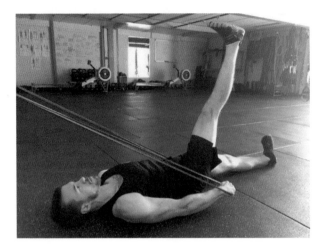

• Lower the leg, return the arms to vertical and repeat the process with the other leg or again with the same leg.

• Repetitions work well in the 10-15 rep range for each leg.

Single Leg Bridge

• The single leg bridge is an excellent exercise to discover asymmetries within the front of the hips and also the abilities of individual glutes to fire. It is also very useful in engaging the glute medius without the larger muscles of the glute taking over the movement.

• Laying on your back, using one leg bridge up firing your glute as hard as you can. Try to avoid using back hyperextension through your lumbar to gain mobility in the exercise. Thighs should remain in line throughout the movement

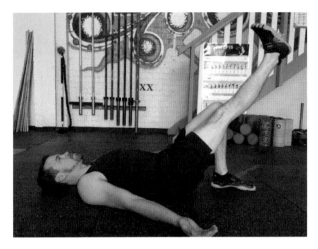

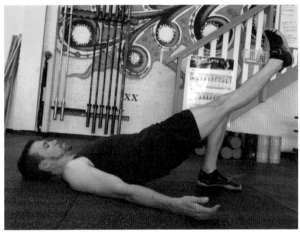

- A more advanced version of this exercise is the Cook Hip Lift created by Gray Cook, this version of the single leg bride helps remove the chance of back hyperextension occurring during the movement by pinning a ball against your abdomen or base of your chest with your raised leg.

- Another traditional form of this exercise is the double leg bridge.

Partnered Hip Activation

- One partner lies on the floor in a supine position.

- Then they bring their legs up to a 90 degrees at the knees and in a vertical femur position.

- The partner then takes hold of the outside of their feet and attempts to pull the feet away from the body.

- Efforts should be made to resist this.

- A short burst of 3-5 seconds is used and then the partner on their back is to rest.

- Repeat this process 5-6 times.

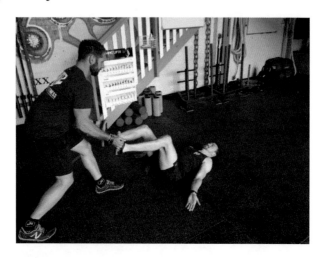

When dealing with positioning of the legs, knees should be open to a point close to resembling the squat, knees should not be held together at any stage.

Squat Prying

- The client is to squat down to the level so that his/her upper legs are parallel with the floor.

- In a normal squat stance (feet just outside shoulder width apart with toes on a 30-45 degree turn out) put the elbows in contact with the inner thigh.

- Forcing the elbows out, the knee will then push outwards, keep the force pushing the knees out.

- From here, rock side-to-side remaining weighted on the heels to prevent overloading the knees with a big chest and shoulders back.

• Continue this for 2-3min only resting when form cannot be maintained.

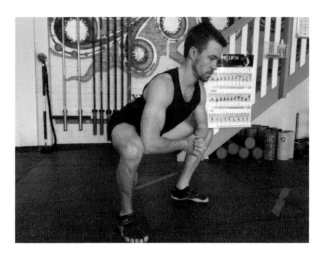

Half Kneeling Hip Flexor with Dowel

• In a half kneeling position, place a dowel in both hands at arms distance.

• Do not become disconnected from your body and maintain an upright position from the downed knee to the head.

• Activating your glute on the downed knee, force the dowel through the floor.

• The hands do not move and the body remains in a vertical position.

• Ensure your hips do not move forward and backwards.

• Maintain tension in the glute and dowel for 5 seconds, relax and repeat 10 times per leg.

Brett Turley

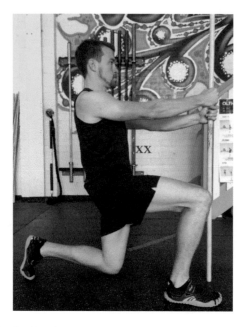

Posterior Chain Activation

•   Squatting down into a position where you can place your hands under your feet set your lats into place by sucking your shoulders to your hips.

•   Maintain a neutral spine throughout the movement, rest when you cannot maintain the correct position.

•   Once your hands are placed under your feet and your lats are set, standup leading with the hips, weighted on your heels.

•   If you have maintained the correct position you will not be able to extend your legs fully and you will feel the stretch through your hamstrings.

•   The idea is to complete this for 2-3 minutes, rest as needed but try and increase movement every repetition.

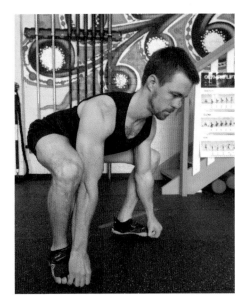

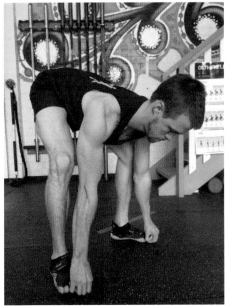

This is a version of Proprioceptive Neuromuscular Facilitation or PNF. The idea is to add resistance through the range of motion or in a static position within a movement pattern creating positional awareness. This will force muscle spindles to lengthen and proprioception will occur, increasing mobility over the period of the movement and improving body awareness.

Brett Turley

RNT is also a version of PNF but more on that later.

Toe Touch

• Placing your heels up onto a plank or board, reach your hands to the sky, shoot your hands down close to your body and try to touch your toes.

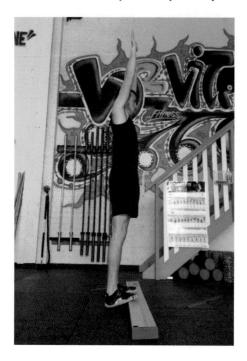

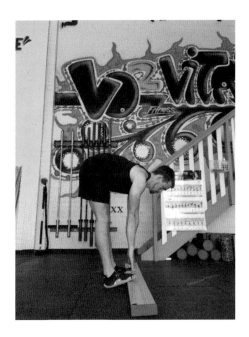

• Repeat this process 10 times and then switch to toes up on the board.

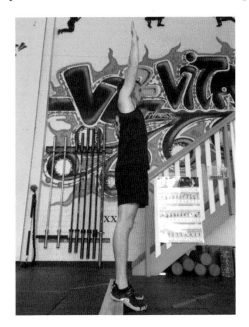

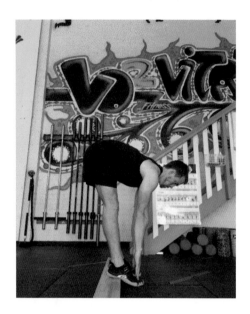

• Keep your knees locked at all times and do not sweep your arms in a wide arc away from the body, keep them close and shift your weight to your heels.

Caterpillars

• These are also referred to as inchworms.

• After reaching up to the sky, shoot the hands down close to the body and touch your toes similar to the toe touch method.

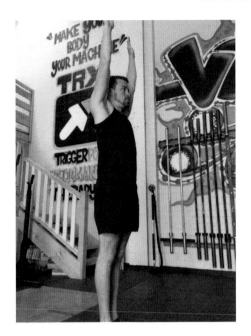

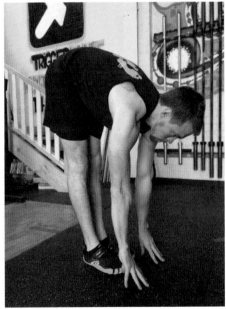

• You are then to walk your hands out all the way to a push-up position maintaining a strong plank position at the finish.

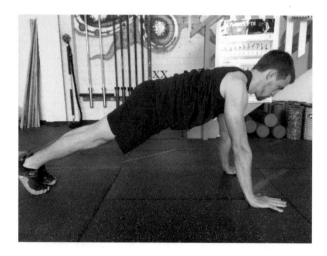

- Following the push-up walk out, pike your hips to the roof and walk your feet back to your hands.

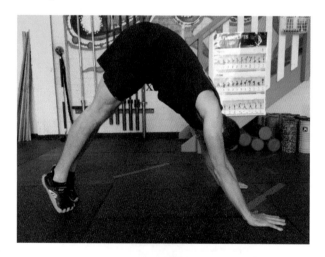

- You can also add a push-up into the sequence if need be.

- Shifting the weight onto each foot as you are bringing your feet to your hands will help you get your feet closer to your hands.

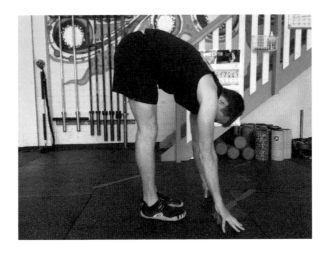

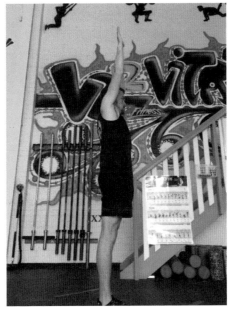

Brett Turley

Shoulders

The shoulder corrective and exercise section encompasses, scapular, thoracic, lat and rotator cuff drills that will keep your shoulders in good health. These exercises should help you gain good mobility and keep your shoulders in the correct and safe position when performing movements or exercise. The ideal position of the shoulders for safe movement is depressed and retracted or down and back, maintaining this is essential to prevent injury.

Wall Sit & Reach

This is a great drill for thoracic mobility.

- Place yourself against a flat wall. Hips should be in contact with the wall at all times with your legs resting on two foam rollers or adequate substitutes if needed.

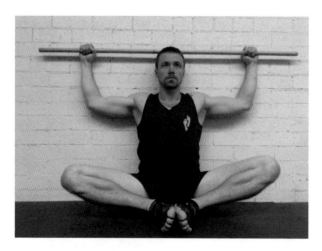

- With the dowel placed on your head and your elbows at 90 degrees, raise your arms up with the wrists and forearms remaining in contact with the wall at all times.

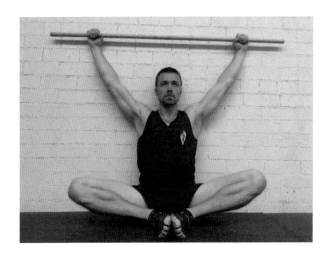

- The drill finishes the moment your wrists and forearms peel away from the wall.

- Complete this exercise for 2-3minutes.

External Rotations

This dowel work does wonders for your rotator cuff and helps activate the smaller, deeper muscles of the shoulder before any heavy pressing or pulling, especially overhead work.

- Grab the end of the dowel in one hand with just enough of the end poking out to see it.

- Leave your other hand open for the dowel to slide through.

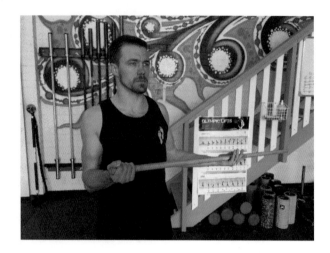

- Keeping your elbow locked in beside your body and your shoulder depressed and retracted (down and back) externally rotate the dowel.

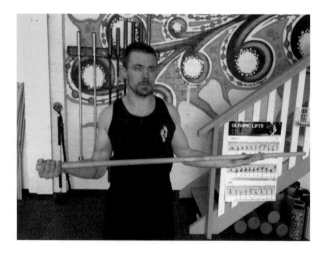

- Continue this until you feel the shoulder warming up, once you can feel the shoulder and rotator cuff activating, complete 5-10 repetitions more and then switch.

Dislocates

The next stage to our shoulder savers is the dislocate.

- Grabbing a wide grip on the dowel engaging the midsection and shoulders (down and back), smoothly pass the dowel over the head without the elbows bending.

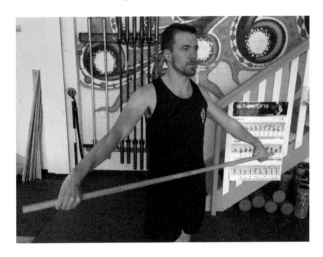

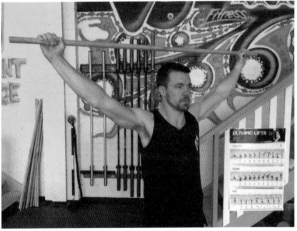

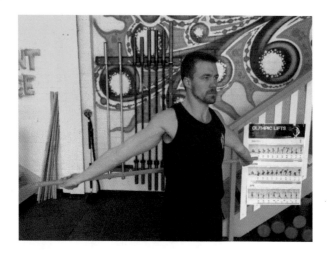

- Without the tension leaving from between the shoulder blades pass the dowel back to the starting point over the head.

- Continue this for 1-2 minutes.

Back Bridge Transition

- Putting yourself into a quadruped stance, transition over so only one hand is in contact with the floor and the other is placed on the hip.

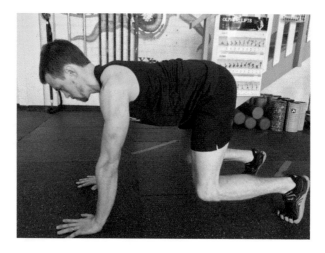

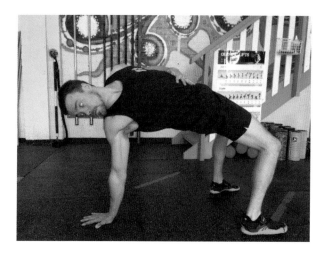

- Keeping focus on your grounded hand, arch your hips to the roof also keeping your rhomboids contracted during the movement.

- Hold this transition period for 30 seconds and switch to the other side.

- Emphasis is placed on keeping your shoulder engaged, eyes on your hand and your hips pushed to the roof.

Halos

- Grabbing a kettlebell of a manageable weight start in the bottoms up position with your hands around the horns and the bottom of the bell at your chin height.

Brett Turley

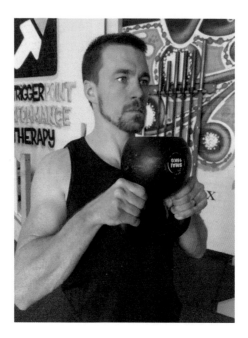

- Once you are set up slowly pass the bell around the back of your head with keeping your head perfectly still.

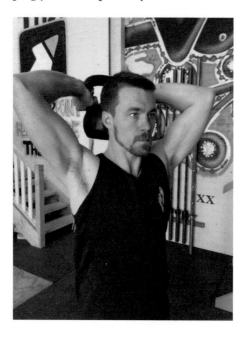

- Catchwords I use are bell around the head, not head around the bell.

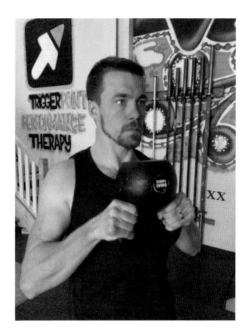

- Sharp breath in through the nose before your start and short breath out as you finish each rep.

- Complete these 10 repetitions each side.

- You can also do this in a half kneeling position to add a challenge for hip stability and shoulder mobility.

Y, T, W, X

You will need an exercise ball or suitable alternative like a bench to facilitate this scapular setting drill. This is probably one of the best drills for the shoulder in this book.

- Once you are set on the exercise ball with your feet against the wall, do 5 repetitions of each letter.

- Be sure to relax your shoulders forward to reset them (protract and then retract and depress) every single rep.

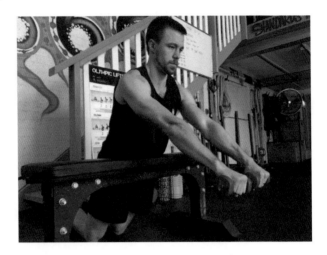

- Start position

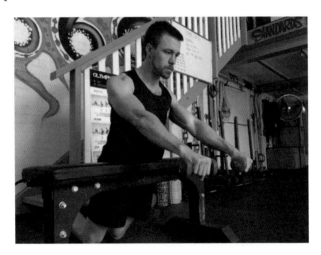

- Y

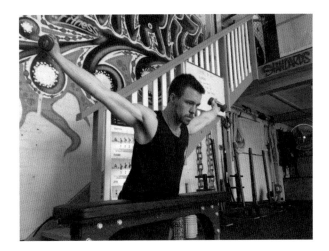

- T

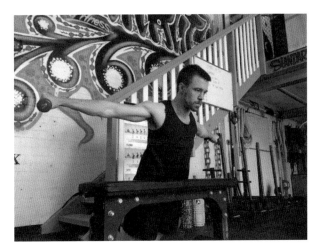

- W – when conducting the "W" on the return to the start position keep your rhomboids engaged as far forward as you can.

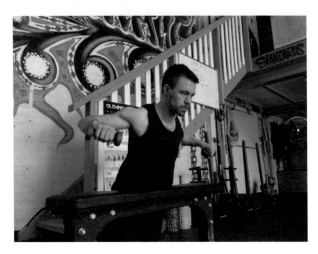

- X – When your wrists bend back on the "X" pattern you have lost shoulder integrity. Avoid letting this happen and maintain a straight wrist through out.

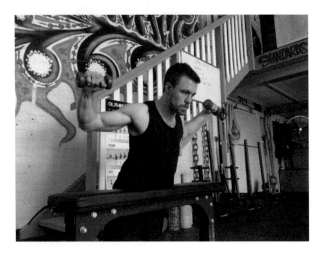

Scapular Setting with Band

- Using a resistance band of low resistance, lock your elbows and triceps placing them parallel to the ground.

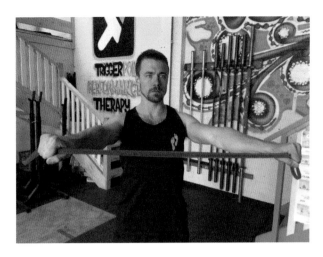

- Pull the band apart without letting your elbows bend and focus on pulling your shoulder blades together with your shoulders down and back.

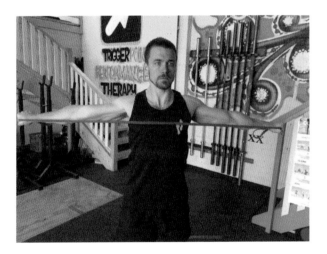

- Repeat this for 10-15 repetitions.

Handstand Holds

- Using a wall to maintain balance practice getting you shoulders into the correct position while holding a handstand.

- Suck your chest to the floor and your shoulders to your feet.

- Keep the glutes engaged as if you were trying to fold them around to your belly button.

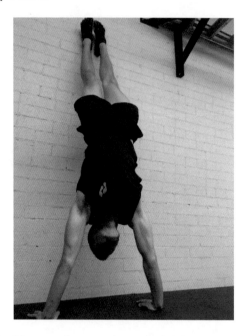

- Hold this for 30 seconds to 1 minute and do 3 repetitions.

Active Hang & Lateral Hang

The active hang involves setting your shoulders from a hanging position.

- Pulling your shoulders to the floor and your chest to the bar, set your shoulder and hold for 30 seconds to 1 minute.

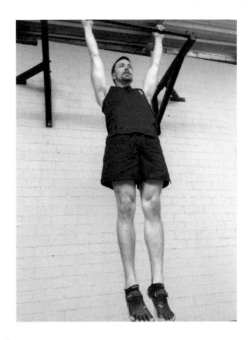

- Work for a few sets.

- Keep your neck relaxed at all times.

- The lateral hang involves engaging the lats to pull you to one side while hanging on the bar.

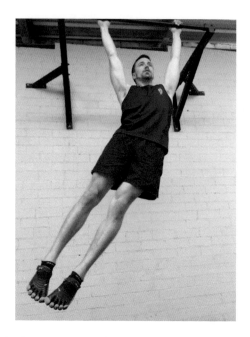

- Without swinging return to the central position and move to the other side.

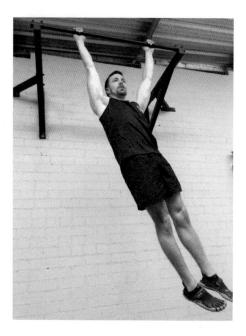

- Do not use your body's momentum to achieve the position.

- Complete 10 lateral hangs on each side.

Arm Bar

Using a kettlebell of a relative weight, 16kg for males and 12kg for females roll over on one side with the kettlebell inline with your stomach.

- Rolling over onto your back with the kettlebell arms elbow remaining in contact with the ground push the opposite leg straight and press the kettlebell up.

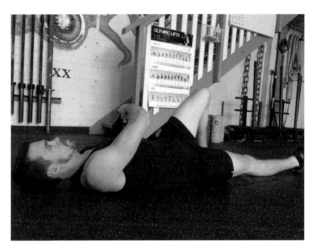

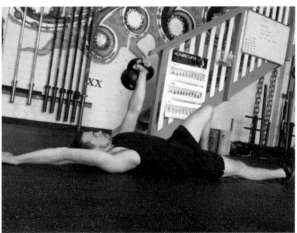

- Bring your opposite arm next to your ear.

- Using your bent leg, raise your hips and the kettlebell into the air until your weight shifts as to place the leg over your other hip to counter balance, stretch the leg out.

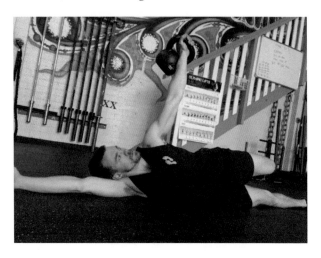

- Your eyes remain on the kettlebell until you are set into position.

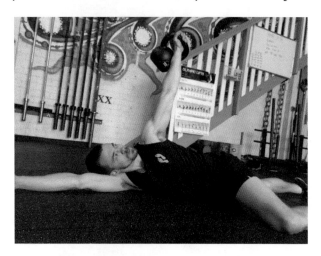

- Once you have set your lat and sucked your shoulder to your hip, take your eyes away from the kettlebell resting your ear on your bicep. Maintain eye contact if you are not confident.

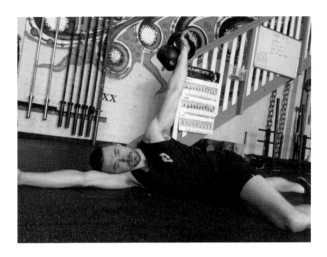

- Once the kettlebell is stable conduct 10 slow breaths into the bottom of your stomach and then reverse in the opposite motion that you came from, placing the bell back onto the floor safely.

- Do this each side for 10 slow breaths.

- Reduce the weight of the bell if necessary to maintain perfect form.

Arm Bar +

- Getting into the arm bar position and engaging your lat (shoulder to hip) start to lower the kettlebell slowly down behind your back keeping your forearm vertical at all times.

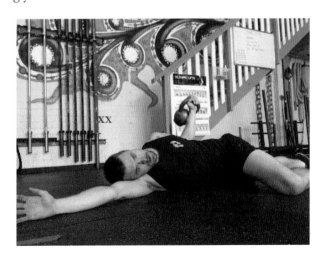

- Conduct ten slow breaths on each side.

- Leave the weight to around 4-12kg and no more.

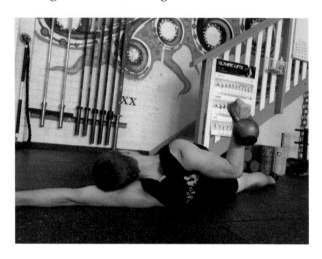

- Be careful if you have had rotator cuff injuries in the past and ensure you have been cleared to use this mobility drill.

Cat Stretch

- In a quadruped position arch your back to the roof.

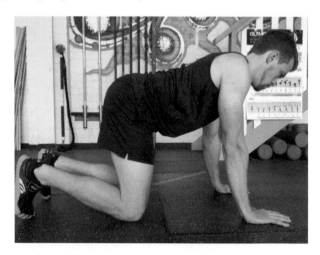

- Imagine someone is giving you a sternum rub on the upper section of your sternum and push yourself away from it.

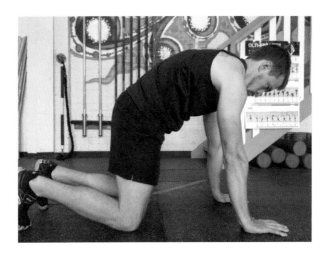

- Hold position for 15-30 seconds and repeat three times.

Ankle & Wrists

Quite often forgotten about in the world of mobility and warm ups, ankle and wrist mobility can drastically improve your performance.

When talking in terms of ankle mobility this has a huge effect on your squat pattern and running style that will keep you away from some of the fundamental issues or injury risks that people face in these exercises particularly at a beginner level.

Ankle Mobility

- In a half kneeling position, place the arm on the inside of the knee but outside of the foot.

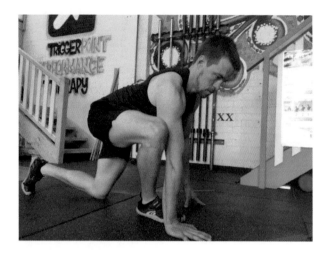

- With the heel remaining in contact with the ground at all times push the knee forward and over the toes and return to starting position.

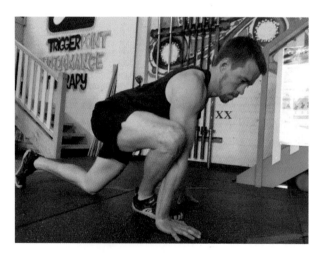

- The moment the heel peels up off the floor you have gone to far, heel must stay planted and the balls of the foot and toes are to stay flat on the ground.

- Repeat sequence for 2-3 minutes each leg.

Wrist Mobility

There are two sections to wrist mobility.

- For the first stage place the back of your hands flat on the floor.

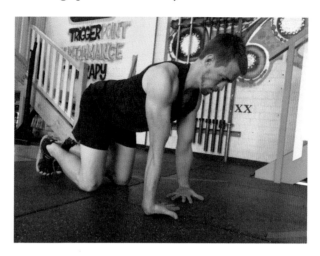

- Keeping your elbows locked, create a fist with the hands and release. Repeat this sequence for 2-3 minutes.

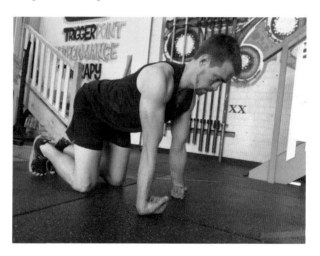

- This will commonly release the trigger points on the back of the wrist that kettlebells sit on when pressing or holding in the rack position.

- Stage two, fingers point back towards the body with the palms flat on the floor.

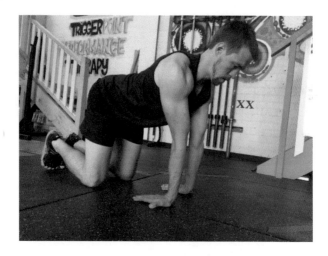

- You are then to bend at the elbows, going into the stretch as far as you can go, pausing for a second and then returning to the start point.

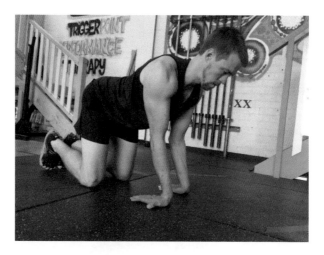

- Repeat this for 2-3 minutes.

Core/Mid-Section

Quadruped Rock with Core Activation

- A resistance band of a medium resistance or exercise ball will be required for this exercise.

- In a quadruped position, place the resistance band over the crease of your glutes and hamstrings to prevent the band from shifting position.

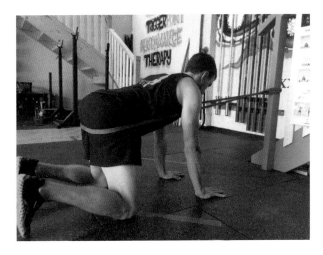

- Pushing away from the anchor point of the resistance band, gain enough tension as to feel like the band is going to pull you forward.

- From here, bracing through the use of diaphragmatic breathing and the mid section, raise one arm with out being pulled off balance.

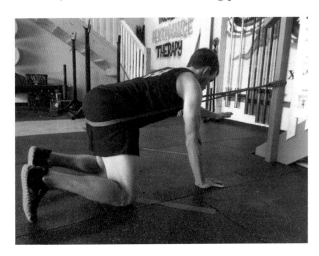

- Return the hand to the floor and repeat with opposing hand.

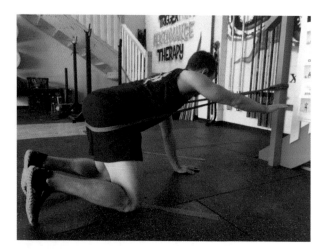

- Repeat for 10 reps each arm.

Bird Dog

For this exercise you will require two resistance bands of equal resistance.

- In a quadruped position, loop a resistance band around each leg and hold on to the bands with the hands.

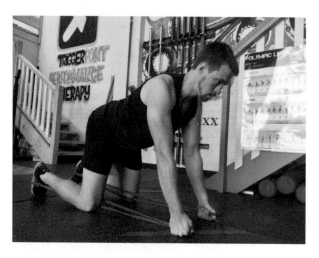

- Now, using reciprocal patterning (opposite limbs moving at the same time) extend one arm and the opposite leg ensuring that the elbow and knee of the extending limbs are locked.

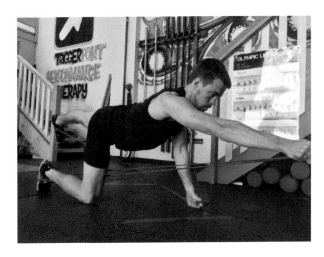

- Repeat for the opposing limbs, 10 repetitions each side.

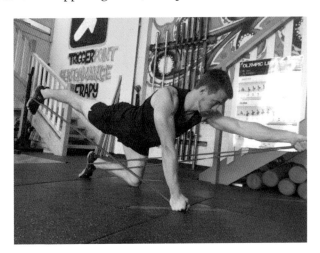

Chop & Lift

This would have to be one of my go to exercises for core activation and coordination between upper and lower body. Utilizing static stability of the hip and dynamic stability of the upper torso this exercise helps coordination in both transverse and sagittal plane exercises.

The Chop –

- Beginning in a half kneeling stance with the inside knee up with your body positioned 45 degrees off the anchor point of the RIP

71

Trainer or resistance band start with hands or handle beside or above the shoulder closest to the anchor point.

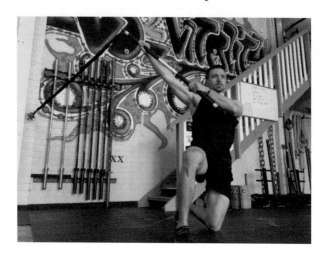

- Pulling through the chest and pushing down and away from the upper body on a 45-degree angle to your hip, maintain your balance and do not let the RIP Trainer or band throw you off balance.

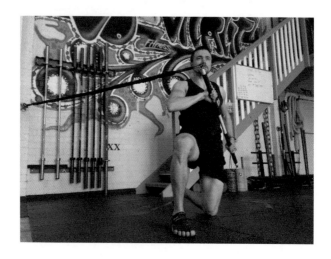

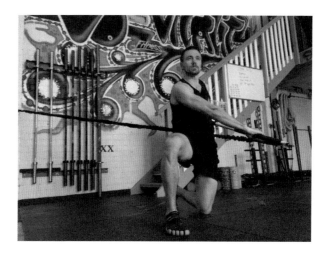

- Keep your glutes and mid section engaged and use a sharp, diaphragmatic breathe to assist the bracing process.

- Release the air through your teeth in a hiss when returning the band or RIP Trainer to the start position.

The Lift – Same principles apply but the outside leg is now up and the start position of the resistance band or RIP Trainer is inline with the hip.

- Pull through the chest and push away from the shoulder at a 45-degree angle.

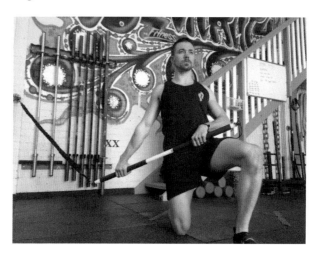

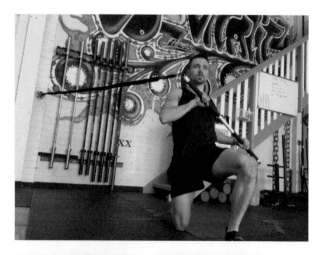

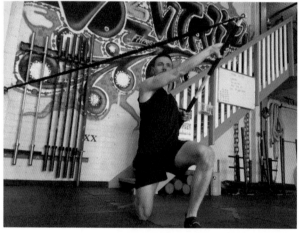

- The same use of bracing and breathing apply.

- Note on the RIP Trainer and resistance Bands – When using the RIP Trainer, hands are in a mid zone position and the hand that is furthest from the anchor point or on the outside utilizes a pulling motion whilst the inside hand pushes, keep the outside hand close to the body.

- When using the resistance band, both hands are placed on the band with the inside hand on the band first being the dominant or driving hand.

- Conduct 10 reps each side for each movement.

Hardstyle Plank

- The exercise was taught to me during my RKC, I haven't found many better exercises to teach people the relation of total body tension required when using kettlebells or performing maximal type lifts due to its ease to teach and queue.

- This is partnered exercise that requires one person to start in the plank position.

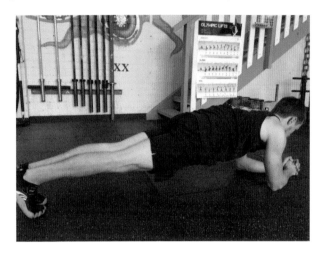

- Following this, the other partner is to tap the lats, abs, glutes and quads of the planking partner, once these muscles have been engaged the partner then gets the planking person to push their feet against their hands with an even amount of force.

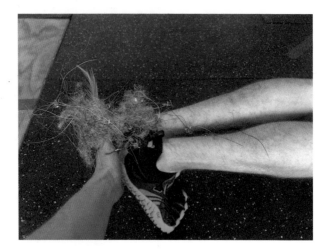

- Hold this for up to 30 seconds.

The muscles to engage are:

Lats: best queue I have used is sucking your shoulders to your hips. Make sure they are not arched through their thoracic region also.

Abs: Midsection is braced using a sharp diaphragmatic breath.

Glutes: Activate your glutes as if you were trying to fold them around to your belly button.

Quads: Suck your kneecaps into your quads and pull your groin or adductors together.

Single Leg Push-up

- The simple single leg push-up is great from mid-section coordination particularly for women learning to keep braced during full push-ups.

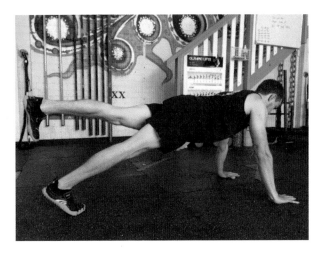

- One leg remains straight or the knee is bent at 90 degrees with the upper leg remaining next to each other during the movement.

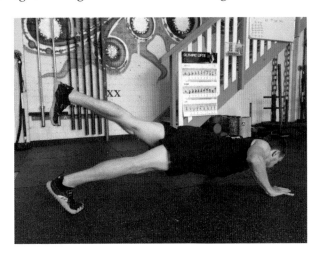

- Perform 5-10 reps with each leg raised.

Get Up

The mother of all mobility and corrective exercises.

Tri-planar, multiple movement patterns are utilized when conducting a correct get up. I don't think there is a more beautiful move when using kettlebells. If you can get up half your bodyweight if you're a male and 24kg for a female, chances are you have covered your mid section/core work and need to look else where for the problem.

- Beginning on one side with the kettlebell inline with your stomach, roll over onto your back with the kettlebell elbow remaining in contact with the ground.

- Set your bent leg off the centre line of the body, in a strong position.

- This position may vary to the individual, as this is your driving leg and glute.

- The out stretched leg is 30-45 degrees off the driving leg creating enough gap between the two.

- The kneecap is sucked into the quad and the toes are pulled back.

- Pressing the bell up with two hands, lock the bell above the chest keeping the shoulder in contact with the ground and the lat activated.

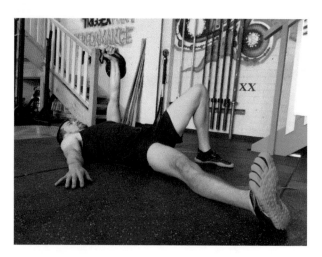

- The outstretched arm runs parallel to the outstretched leg.

- Using a sharp abdominal breath and eyes remaining on the bell at all times, drive up off your bent leg whilst activating your glute over to your other side being sure not to try and just sit up, the moment you feel your weight shift over to your opposite elbow drive it into the ground and get tall.

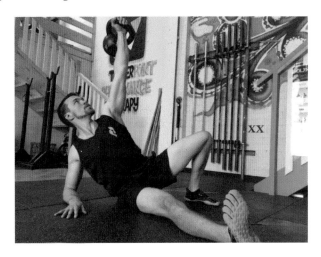

- Joints should be stacked from the grounded elbow all the way up to the wrist holding the kettlebell.

- From here, pivoting on your hand, turn your fingers out and come up into your tall sitting position off your elbow.

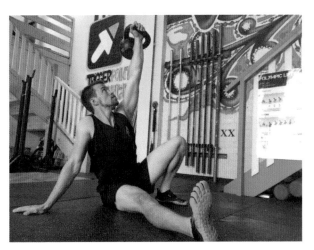

- Do not move the hand, just pivot on it.

- From your tall sitting position push your hips off the ground into the low bridge position.

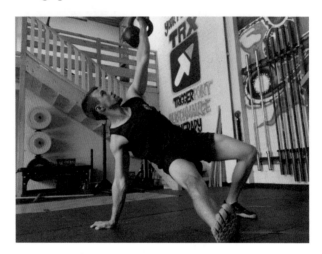

- From your low bridge, conduct your leg sweep of the outstretched leg underneath yourself until the femur is vertical and supporting your weight.

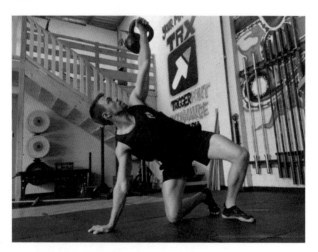

- Hand should be in line with the knee and the foot in a side kneeling position.

- From the side kneeling position, come up to a half kneeling position with the hand off the ground utilizing your hip hinge pattern.

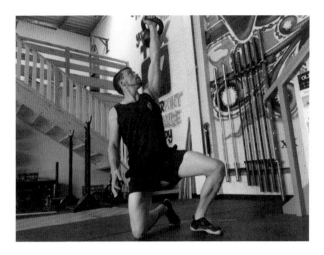

- Eyes will then come forward.

- Windshield wiper the back foot into an inline half kneeling stance.

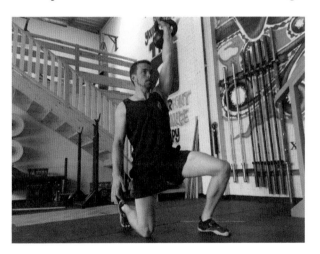

- Parting the floor with both feet drive straight up standing tall finishing with feet shoulder width apart.

Brett Turley

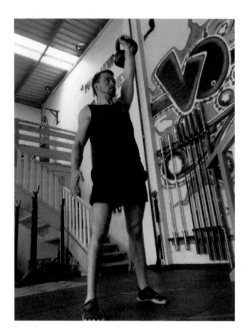

- Reverse the process to return to the start position.

Back Body Line Drill

Huon and Petra Feitscher taught the next two bodyline drills to me from Kudos Gym in Sydney. These have an awesome carry over for overhead pressing and holds. For this exercise you will need a dowel and a small 1.25kg weight or equivalent.

- Laying on your back place the dowel above your chest with the weight centred, pretending to snap the dowel to gain tension on it.

- You legs are raised together with your toes pointed to the roof and your quads and adductors tight.

- Your lower back is pushed into the ground and your glutes and abs are engaged.

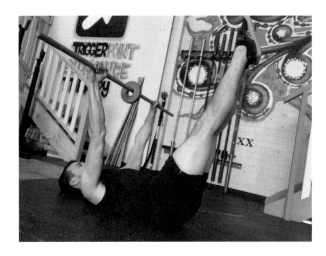

- From here, lower your legs and arms to the floor keeping elbows locked, tension on the dowel toes pointed.

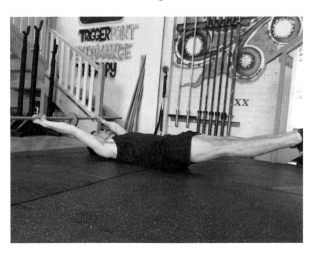

- Lower down until just before the lower back starts to peel up off the floor the aim is to finish just above the floor with the arms and legs.

- The weight or feet should not hit the floor at any time.

- To help get the most out of the exercise you can have someone lightly punching your abdominals or for the advanced have someone standing on your abdominals during the movement, do not try this until you have perfected it.

- The lower back should remain in contact with the floor at all times during the movement.

- Practice this drill; there are no set repetitions, as this will be quite taxing.

Front Body Line Drill

- Laying on your stomach, plantar flex or point your toes away from your body, fold your hips around to your belly button forcing them into the floor.

- Push your stomach into the floor the same as your chest.

- Your nose stays just in contact with the floor.

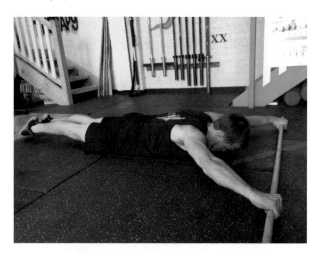

- This can be done with your hands out in a crucifix position with fists clenched fingers facing the floor to begin or with a dowel above your head with elbows locked similar to a snatch grip. Hold for up to 30 seconds and repeat only a couple of times.

Loaded Carries

We have three traditional types of carries that we can utilize they are in order from easiest to most difficult.

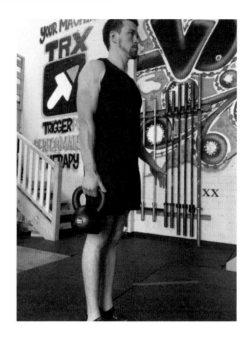

Farmers,

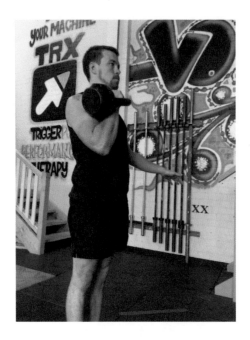

Rack and:

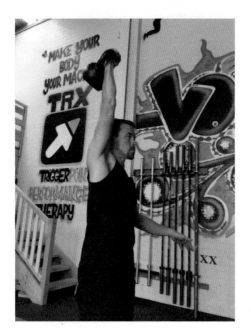

Overhead.

These can be done with single or double kettlebells and are great for teaching breathing under tension and anterior core activation. Set your distance and repeat as much as needed. These can be placed anywhere with in your workout but do not load excessively during the warm up. Stay tight and "breath behind the shield" as it's said.

Asymmetrical Presses & Carries

Single sided or asymmetrical loading exposes a lot of issues on individual sides of the body. When asymmetries are within the body this increases the injury risk by up to 3.5 times. Asymmetrical exercises include:

- The above loaded carries with a single bell,

- Pressing varieties with a kettlebell particularly the floor press for core activation and;

- Single leg work.

<u>Patterning</u>

- This brings all of your MCT, mobility and core work together. Many of these drills have multiple effects with in the movement patterns such as asymmetrical work but emphasis is placed on whole movement patterns or whole body exercises.

- Great from warm ups as they challenge mobility and motor control putting a higher neural and physical load on the body.

- When trying to gain good movement, keep the repetitions small and avoid fatigue until competency is acquired.

Rolling

Soft Rolling –

- This can be done by upper and lower body; you can also use assistance such as foam rollers underneath your body to help initiate the rolling pattern.

- These are great exercises to use during work sets or to even wind down after training.

- They are neurologically challenging and have a tonic effect to calm you down after a big session.

- These are developmentally the basis for all patterning as we learn to do this when we are babies learning how to move our bodies for the first time.

- The respective limbs initiate upper and lower body soft rolling, effort is made to relax the rest of the body to allow the moving limbs to initiate and carry out the roll.

Here are some examples of soft rolling:

Upper Body:

- Laying supine or on your back use the head to initiate the roll by placing it over the shoulder in the way you are rolling, the arm will then follow suit coming across the body reaching over as far as possible as to pull the rest of the body across.

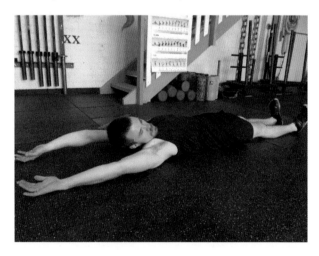

- Eyes are on the moving hand to emphasize the pull across.

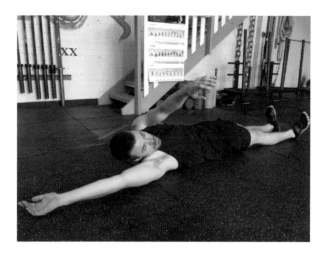

- The arm will then shoot back above the head pulling the body across over to a prone position.

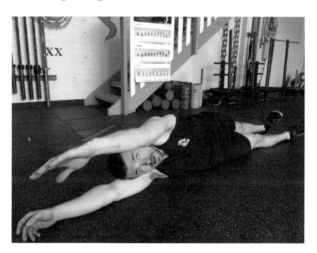

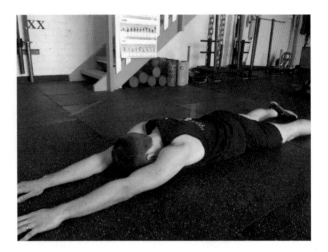

- From the prone position the arm sweeps back over the body with the eye firmly fixed and following the moving hand.

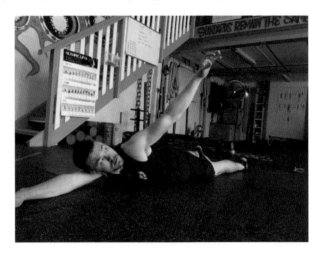

- The moving arm is then used to extend as far as possible engaging the pull back across onto the back.

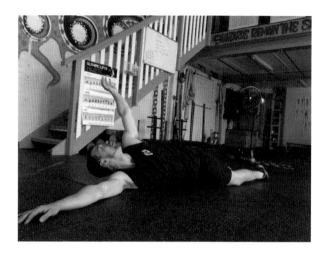

- The arm will then shoot back above the head finishing the roll.

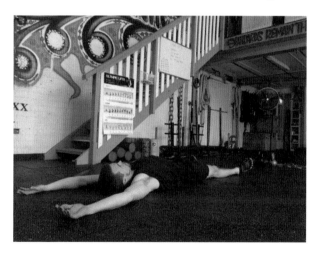

Lower Body: initiated with the legs in a supine position, the leg is brought up with the bent knee and pulled across to the other side.

- The knee is pulled far enough to bring the hip up off the ground and to start the weight shifting.

Brett Turley

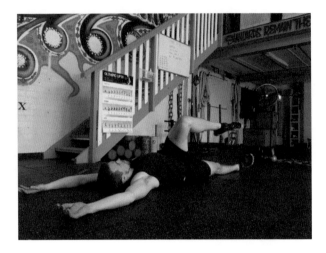

- The leg is then pushed back out to an extended position pulling the body over to prone.

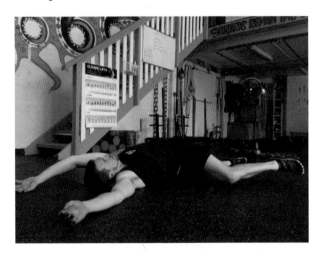

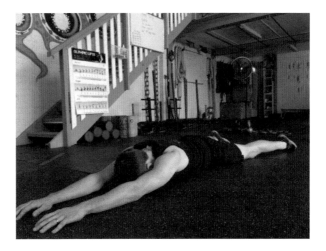

- To initiate the roll back over to supine, the knee is bent and pulled across the body with the foot reaching out as far as possible to start the roll.

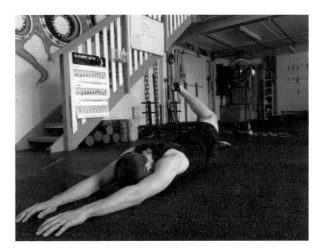

- Once the centre of mass starts to shift the leg is extended pushing the foot back out and finishing the roll.

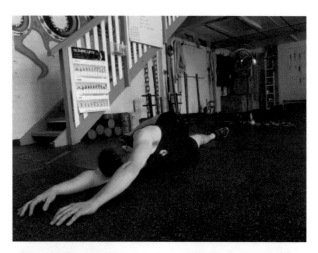

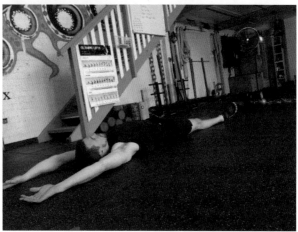

- After you have achieved competency in soft rolling we can progress this to hard rolling. Often very difficult to teach and initiate with people this will challenge coordination and core control and the movement is initiated with the head only.

Rocking

- Another great exercise to use between work sets as this helps free up the hips in preparation for squatting or similar movements and also shows that someone has adequate mobility for the squatting pattern among other benefits.

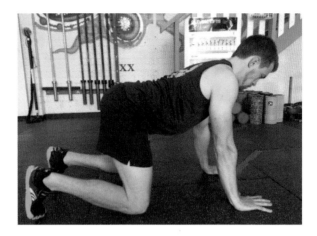

- In a quadruped position rock back and forth sitting deep into the squat pattern.

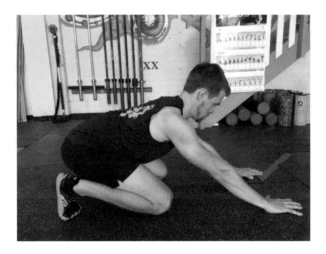

- You can also utilize a head tilt both front and back to clear up the pattern show people the ideal head and spine position during a squat.

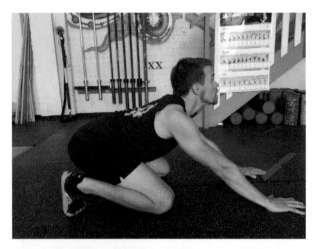

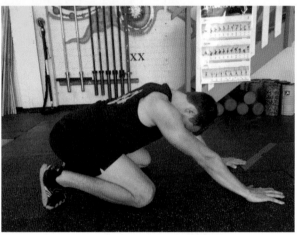

Crawling

As children we used to spend a lot of time crawling before we learned how to walk and eventually began reducing activity and sitting around in chairs with poor posture and switching off.

- Crawling is a great way to wake up the neurological pathways to better movement and can be used as a conditioner on itself due to its inefficient nature.

- To begin crawling you must ensure that the patterning of the exercise is available to you.

- Reciprocal patterning is the way to go when crawling meaning opposite limbs move at the same time, the same as running.

- You can begin this on your knees.

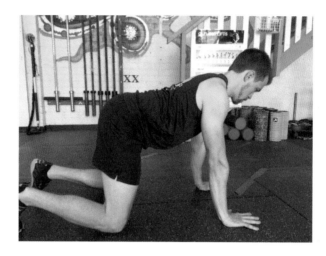

- Moving to knees up with the hips higher than the shoulders are often the next stage as people develop the core strength to maintain this position.

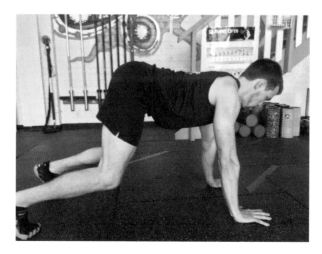

- Once this has been established we then move to a more dynamic posture with the hips lower than the shoulders.

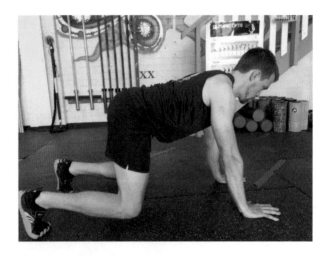

- This will be far more demanding on the body.

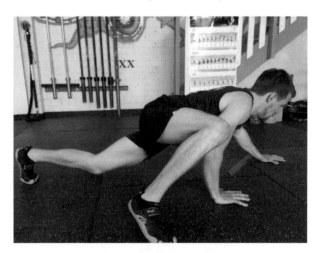

- Crawling backwards or laterally at any of these stages will also challenge the body and mind further.

Squat with RNT

To keep it simple Reactive Neuromuscular Training means to use resistance or an outside influence to pull the limb or movement pattern further into the problem forcing the body to compensate to correct the issue to improve body and positional awareness.

- We can do this within the squat in a variety of manners.

- To stop valgus collapse we can attach a resistance band to the outside of an individual knee or both knees to force compensation outwards to prevent the inwards collapse.

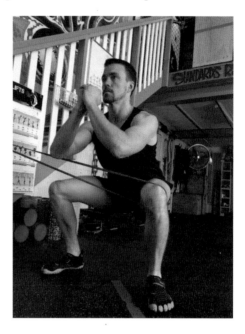

- If the hips shift laterally or fail to load deep enough back into the squat a band can placed to force the correct movement.

- Remember to pull into the problem.

- To help your overhead work, a band can be placed around the shoulders and pulled forward to initiate the body staying upright during the squat.

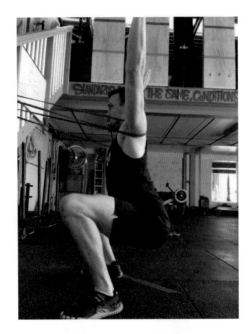

- They can also be placed around the hands pulling forward to assist.

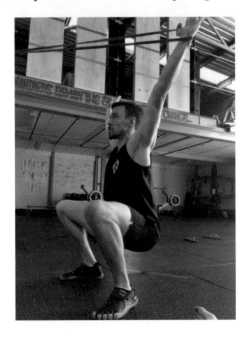

Goblet Squat

Using a kettlebell this could be hands down one of the easiest ways to teach someone how to squat correctly.

- With the hands around the horns of the bell and using it as a counter weight, squat down until full depth is achieved.

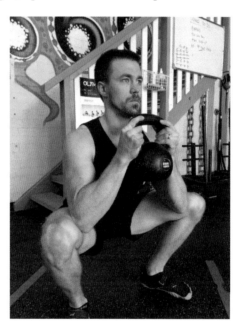

- When coming out of the squat, lead with the shoulders to ensure the weight does not pull you forward while also driving through the heels and engaging the glutes.

Face The Wall Squat

This will test coordination within your squatting pattern and your thoracic mobility.

- Stand as close as you can to a wall and squat down.

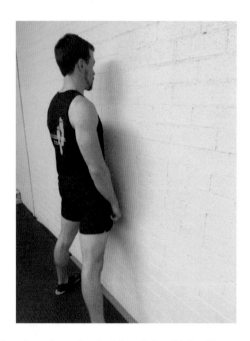

- Hands can be placed on the inside of the thighs like you are picking something up from the floor.

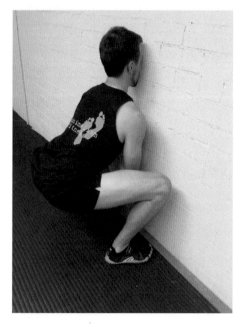

- To add a more difficult progression squat down close to a wall with your hands above your head as if to be in an overhead squat position.

- Ensure the feet do not turn out past 30-45 degrees during the movement.

Lunge with RNT

- In a split stance position, connect a resistance band to the outside of the front knee pulling the knee in to the problem.

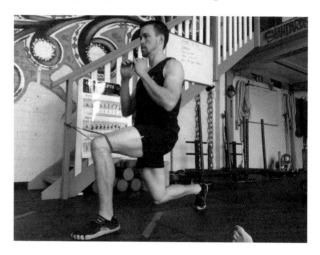

- Conduct a lunge back wards and resist the band pulling you in.

Floor Press

- The floor press is one of my favorite go to exercises when teaching core activation for a strong push-up or press.

- Using the ground to gain feedback or increase proprioception press the kettlebell up from the floor to above your shoulder.

- The lat should stay engaged, the opposite arm should be palms up and your midsection should be tight with the use of diaphragmatic breathing.

- Knees are bent with the feet planted in a comfortable position.

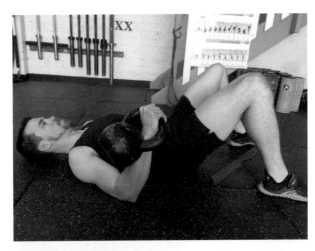

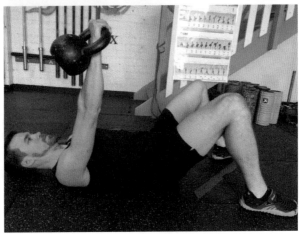

Push-up

Many people, especially females struggle when performing correct push-ups. Normally taught in a high rep scenario focus is based on just churning out the reps regardless of form. If you learn the push-up correctly it can be one of the best upper-body strength builders going around particularly for females.

- Ideally hand should be placed roughly just outside shoulder width apart but still inline with the shoulders.

- Elbows should be tucked in on a 45-degree angle with the lats engaged.

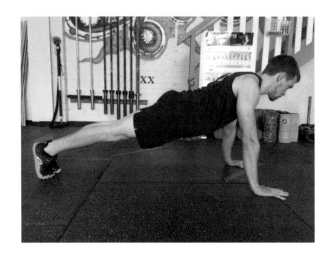

- Instead of focusing on your chest during the push-up, focus on your lats and pulling yourself to the floor.

- When this occurs tension is maintained and the stretch reflex engages to pull you out of the bottom of the push-up.

- Ideally upper-arm should be horizontal at depth. Chest to floor is optimal.

- When pushing out of the bottom, emphasize cork screwing your elbows in, to wind your lats on tightly.

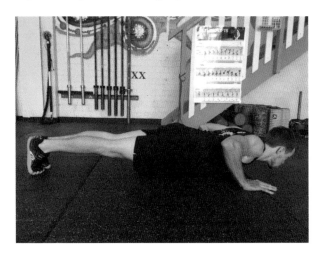

- This should be your focus, this will enable the chest to actually push and your synergist and antagonist muscles to stabilize and support the movement.

- Abs, glutes and quads should be engaged throughout the movement to prevent sagging at the mid section or lower back and diaphragmatic breathing should be utilized.

Bottoms Up Press

This exercise is great for activating your lats and rotator cuff within your press. Having your lats and rotator cuff firing during your press is essential particularly when looking at pressing a new 1 Rep Max (1RM).

- When the bell is on the floor force your hand onto it and grip it tightly.

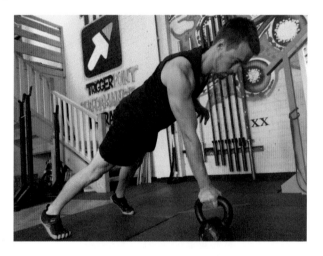

- Do not re-grip throughout the whole movement.

- Ensure you have chalk on your hands when pushing a heavy bell.

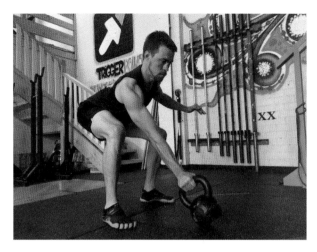

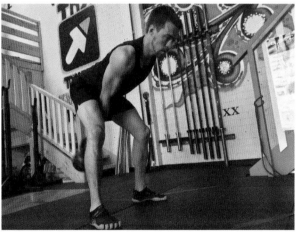

- Without loosening your grip, hike the bell up to a bottom up position with the hand starting underneath the chin.

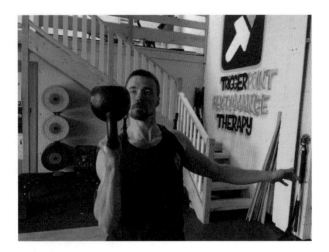

- Keep your lat and glute switched on to lock the bell in place for the starting position.

- With the eyes on the bell and a sharp diaphragmatic breath into the stomach begin to press the bell to a full lock out.

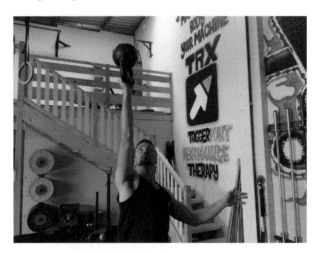

- Emphasize pushing yourself away from the bell rather than pressing it into position.

- Maintain tension throughout and return to the start position still keeping tight.

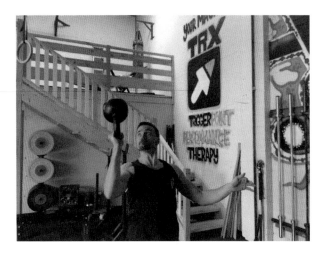

- You can do these with singles or multiple reps. Bottoms up squats and walks are also great lat and rotator cuff builders.

KB Press

- Without the limit of a fixed hand position when using a barbell for pressing, the kettlebell press is a great way to build overhead strength and patterning that allows good range of motion through your thoracic region.

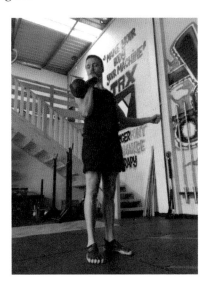

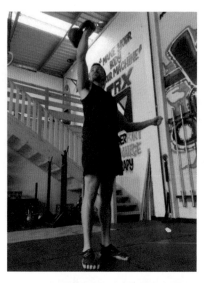

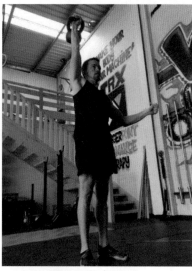

- These can be done a variety of ways such as single, double and alternating.

- See the tips and techniques section for a bigger kettlebell press.

Hip Hinge Patterning

- Done with a dowel on your back with three points of contact being the head, thoracic and sacrum (tailbone) hip hinge patterning will activate your posterior chain and lengthen hamstrings and glutes that are bound up from excessive sitting or little use.

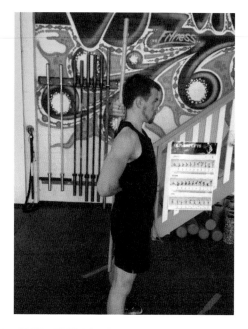

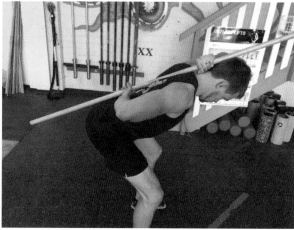

- With the glutes being the strongest muscle group in the human body it is amazing to see so few people using the hip hinge pattern to build a strong and robust physique.

- Conduct the hip hinge patterning exercise for 2-3 minutes pushing into the pattern as deep as possible without letting the three points of contact be lost.

- With the hip hinge remember, shoulders above the hips, hips above the knees at all times.

- For athletic cases developing a strong hip hinge pattern will improve your athletic ability and explosiveness by not relying on the quads to initiate powerful movements in an athletic stance.

Suitcase Deadlift

- This can be done with a barbell or kettlebell and is a form of RNT.

- Using the single sided exercise this will force the body to compensate to brace the core and stay level during the activity.

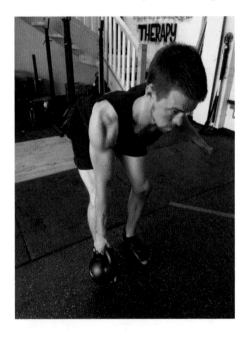

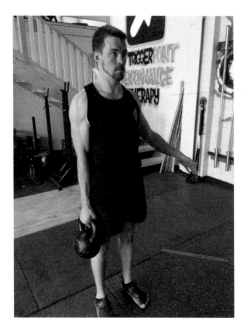

- Conducting a short amount of suitcase deadlifts before heavy deadlifting has seen many improvements in technique and weight with minimal fuss.

Contra lateral Single Leg Deadlift (SLDL)

Another form of RNT using a kettlebell, the SLDL has many carry over effects such as lat activation, core stability and hip hinge patterning. This would be another of my go to correctives for almost anyone.

- When conducting the contra lateral SLDL the kettlebell is in the hand of the moving leg.

- Ipsilateral is the alternative but is usually easier, give both a try.

- Starting with the kettlebell in the hand in a standing position, kick your moving leg back extending through the heel with the toes pointing to the floor.

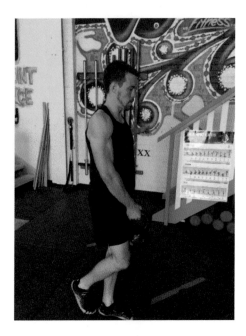

- Emphasis is placed on the heel push to the wall behind you to keep loaded in the hip hinge position to prevent "quadding".

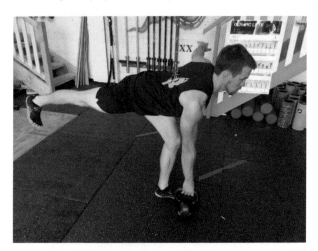

- The lats are activated at all times with the opposite hand counter balancing with the core engaged to prevent dropping at either end.

- As much as the foot moves the shoulders follow until horizontal or just above it reached.

- Do not become disconnected.

- You can advance this exercise by starting with the bell on the floor and moving to it.

- Having to brace mid lift with the bell on the floor will make it more challenging.

- The lighter the bell, the harder the movement.

Kettlebell Swing

- The kettlebell swing, as much as it is regarded as a great conditioning tool is also an excellent corrective.

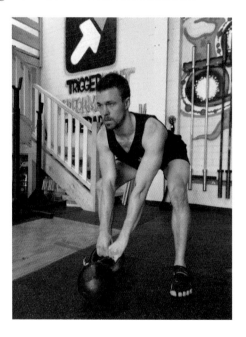

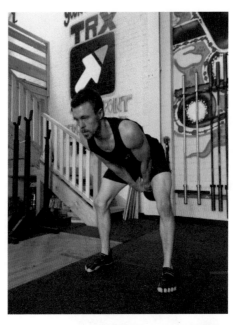

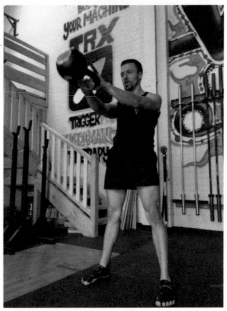

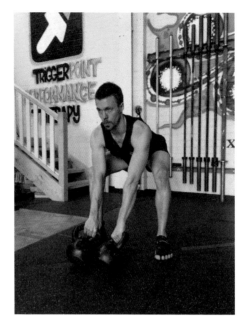

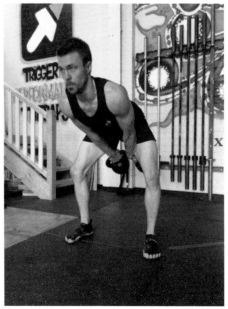

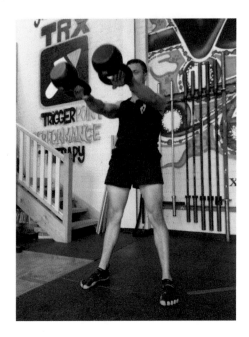

- Similar to the SLDL the kettlebell swing and in particular the single arm swing forces a correct hip hinge pattern, lat activation to pack the shoulder and core coordination for maximum tension and relaxation.

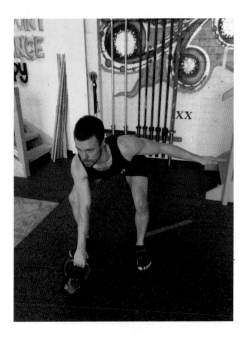

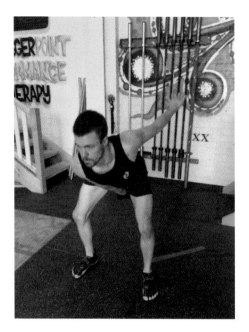

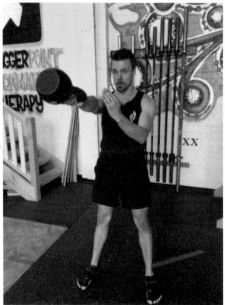

Bat Wing Row

Done on a bench with a small ROM this focuses on a muscle group often
forgotten, the rhomboids.

- Laying face down on a bench with your forehand against it to prevent arching of the back pick up two kettlebells bringing your thumbs to your armpits.

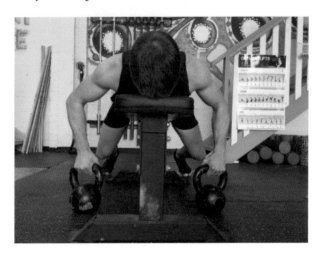

- Squeeze you shoulder blades together focuses on the rhomboids. Shoulders should be packed in the correct position with the lats activated.

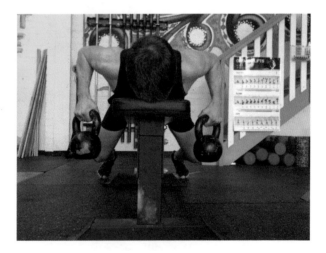

- Repeat for sets of 5, if you feel the cramping between your shoulder blades you are doing it right

Real Row

- The real row starts to bring the full pulling pattern together.

- Requiring a strong position of the spine in a neutral position, core must be used to maintain it.

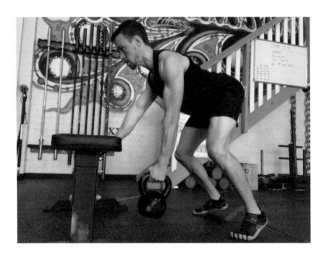

- Keeping up on the balls of the feet also reduces stability from the base of support.

- Row with the elbow and not the shoulder, focus pulling the elbow back until the kettlebell handle is beside the body.

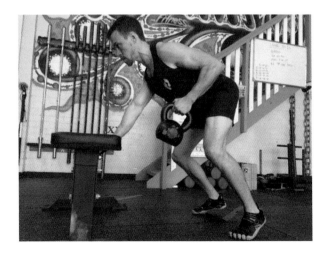

- Shoulder is packed on the opposite arm and the elbow is locked.

Renegade Row

- Starting from a push-up start position, row a kettlebell to your hip.

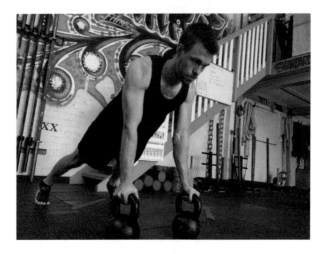

- To help stability push your other hand into the non-moving kettlebell to ground yourself.

- Be sure not to raise your hip to help the row.

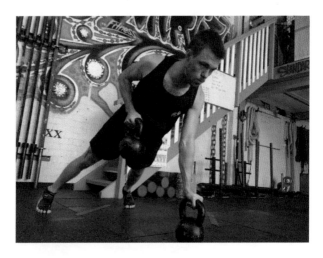

- The feet can be spread wider to help also.

- You can mix in your push-up practice here also, having the kettlebells will raise the incline of your push-up potentially making it easier, grip the bells and cork screw those elbows in to get up out of the bottom position.

- You can also go deeper into a deficit push-up to develop your push-ups further.

5 THE PREHAB PROGRAM

Goal: Become Injury Free

You can choose to do this program two or four days a week. If you are training two days a week, put the single arm swings and get ups in the same session. If you are training four days a week, split them apart onto alternate days, training four days a week would be my recommendation. This program is based from FMS correctives and Pavel's RKC Program Minimum. The focus of the program is perfect form and to progress to a weight that is challenging. Finish weights for the get ups and swings for male and female are:

Male: 32kg

Female: 24kg

You finish the program when you can:

- **Complete 200 single arm swings in 12 minutes with a 24 or 32kg kettlebell and...**
- **Complete 5 Get Ups per side with in 10 minutes with the 24 or 32 kg kettlebell.**

The rest of the exercises are the prehab phase of the program. This prehab program has seen ladies at the ages of 50 and 57 complete a 250km adventure race through the Simpson Desert, seen many individuals become injury and pain free from shoulder injuries and bulletproofed athletes for the beginning of pre-season training for their given sport. So here it is:

Kettlebell Arm Bar – 3/3(L/R) 10 breathes per side

Bear Crawling – 3 minutes

Get Up – 3/3 un-weighted

Single Leg Hip Bridge – 10/10

Halos – 10/10

Goblet Squat – 3x10

Hip Hinge Patterning with dowel – 3 minutes

Chop & Lift – 10/10 each side

Single Leg Deadlift – 10/10

10min - Get Up – 5/5

12min - Single Arm Swings – 10/10 (As Many Sets As Possible)

How do we know when to progress? When the weight feels easy. You are to have one easy day **60-70%** of each main exercise being the Get Up and Swing and one harder day **80-90%** per week. If you are feeling flat, switch the hard day for an easy day. Only push hard and go all out once in a while, just to test where you are. Let the results come by you gently encouraging them. Sticking to this simple program will be a lot harder than what you think, challenge yourself to go the distance and don't give up until you have achieved the master steps.

Brett Turley

6 EVOLUTION OF MAN

Goal: Bodyweight Strength & Mastery

The Evolution of Man is a bodyweight program that will see you develop your ability to steer your own body to levels of strength most others will not be able to do. It is done without any equipment except for the aid of a pull-up bar. This could be your low cost entry in to the Minimalism Effect. It runs for a four-day split, but where you place your four days in your week is up to you. Common splits would be:

Monday, Wednesday, Thursday & Saturday

Monday, Tuesday, Thursday & Saturday

Monday, Wednesday, Friday & Saturday

The aim of the program is to progress through to the most advanced version of the exercise as you can. Progressions and regressions have been supplied for you to work at your own level. Don't forget to use the bulletproofing for your body sections to help with correctives and technique. Here is the tricky part, for all of you *guns* out there; you must start from the beginning of the skills progression.

You have three avenues of approach when it comes to this program. Choose one and stick to it. The three focuses are:

High Volume Basics (push-ups, pull-ups & squats)

- Follow the progressions to full push-ups, pull-ups and squats.

- Stop here and work your consolidation work, on the days given.

- Push the other three progressions for the handstand push-ups, hanging leg raise and bridge, but doing a running and jump day is optional.

- This focus is targeting strength endurance for a beginner level.

Just Skills

- Set out to master all six skills.

- No running or consolidation work.

- Instead of the consolidation work add in extra skill work if you feel you need it.

- For example, consolidation push-ups on day one will become one arm push-up skills progression.

- This will drop you to a 3 day a week program.

- This is targeting someone who is trying to advance above standard bodyweight skills.

The Whole Nine Yards

- Work your skills and consolidation work on the given days.

- Keep the running and jump day in also.

- This is the most advanced method.

- Stick it out until you complete all skills.

- Cycle through your 4 weeks and repeat as necessary.

- If you are having trouble busting through a training plateau, add your consolidation work into your training or visit the breaking

Brett Turley

plateaus section in the training tips.

Weekly Breakdown

1	2	3	4
Pistol Squats	One-Arm Pull-ups	One-Arm Push-ups	Jump
Hanging Leg Raise	Handstand Push-ups	Bridging	Running
Push-ups (C)	Squats (C)	Pull-ups (C)	Nil.

(C) – Consolidation Work
Nil – No Consolidation Work on Day 4

Perform testing for push-ups, squats & pull-ups before starting your program. Testing will allocate you to beginner, intermediate or advanced for consolidation work.

The beauty of this program is the strength work is practice, let the strength come naturally, don't force yourself into thinking that over training will deliver the results you require. Don't forget to read the waving loads section in the training tips to help keep you fresh with minimal plateaus in your training.

The running & jumping progression plan for day 4, runs on a 4-week split of Monday, Wednesday, Friday & Saturday. Emphasis should be placed on technique within this session just like your strength practice. Let the speed come as you focus on skills. The jumping element also requires equipment, due to the complexity of some of the exercises, you can also regress adequately during your training, if you feel fresh enough to do it, go right ahead. If you are progressing to Pistol Squats and you like your hip flexors, they will take one hell of a beating, so take it easy on your running and jump day and conduct an adequate warm up that has a dynamic element.

Skills Progression

Pistol Squat

1. Standard Squat 2x20

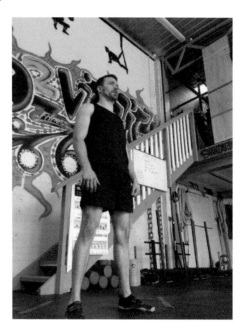

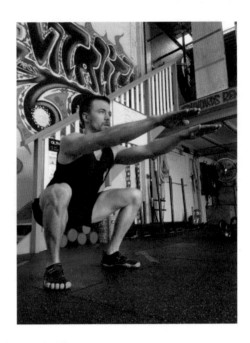

2. Close Feet Squats 2x20

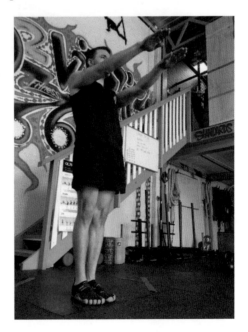

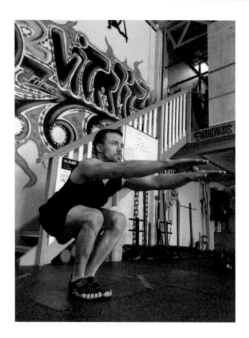

3. Bench Pistol Squat 2x5-10

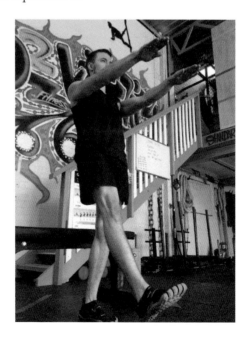

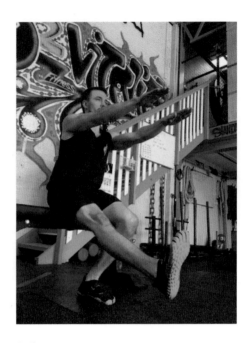

4. Skater Lunge 2x5

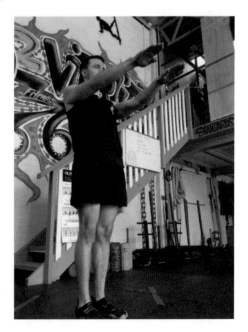

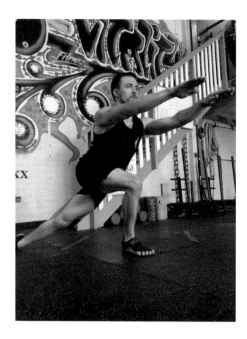

5. Eccentric phase with weight 5x1

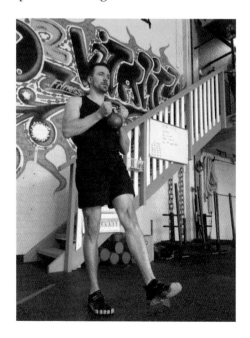

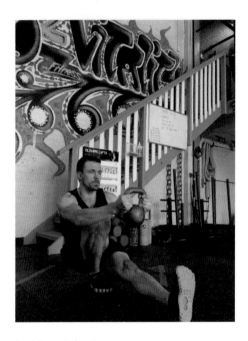

6. Full Pistol with weight 5x1

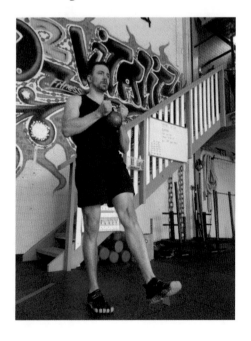

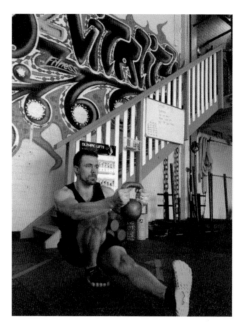

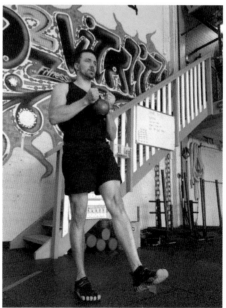

7. Elevated Pistol 5x1

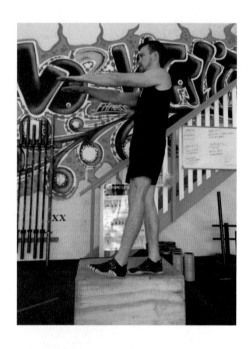

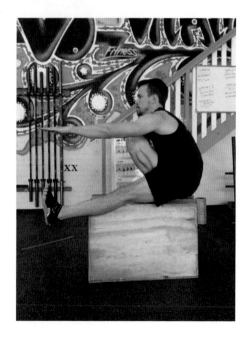

8. Full Pistol Squat

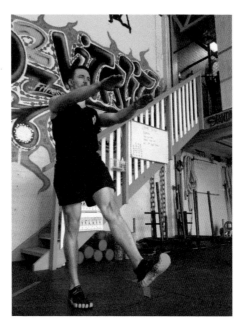

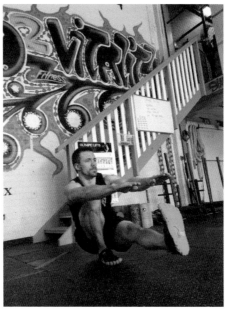

One-Arm Push-up

1. Incline/TRX Push-ups 2x30

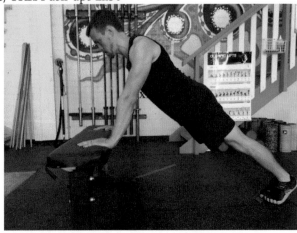

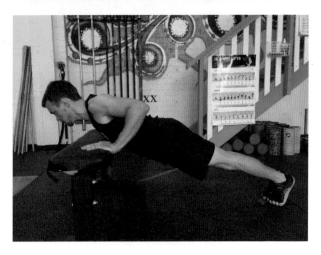

2. Half Push-ups 2x20

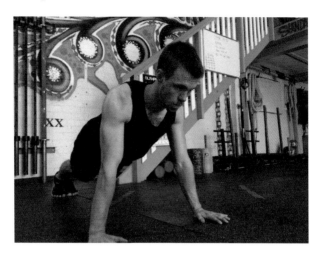

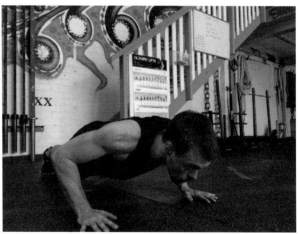

3. Full Push-ups 2x20

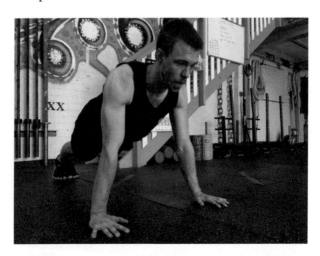

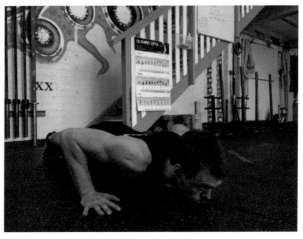

4. Diamond Push-ups 2x10-20

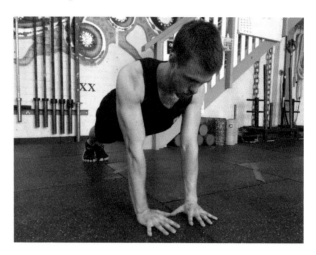

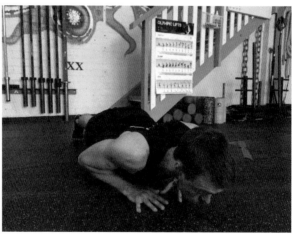

5.   Uneven Push-ups 2x10

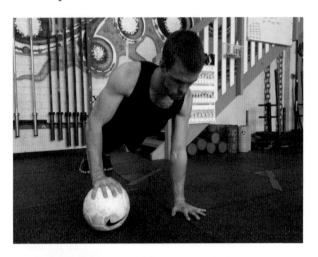

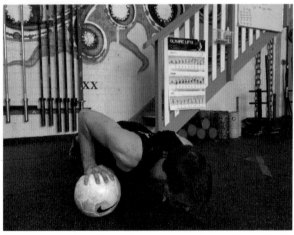

6. Elevated One-Arm Push-ups 2x5

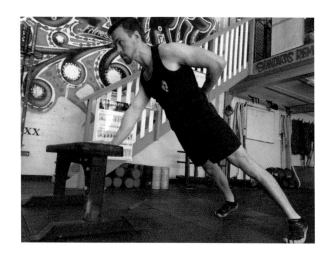

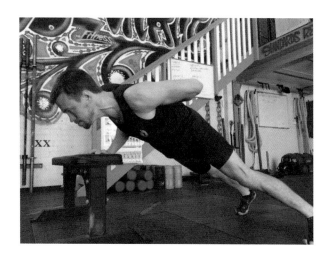

7. Lever Push-ups 2x5

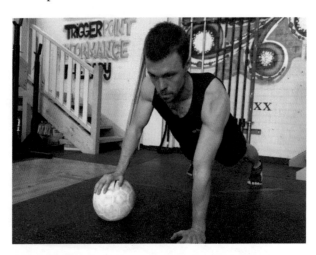

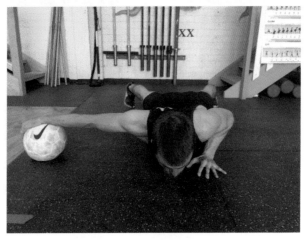

8. **One-Arm Push-up**

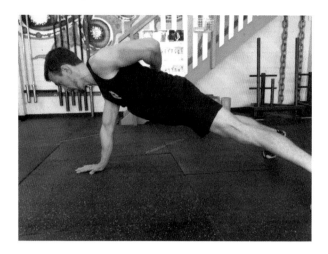

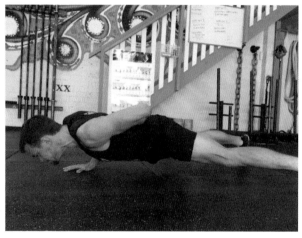

One-Arm Pull-up

1. Inverted Row 2x30

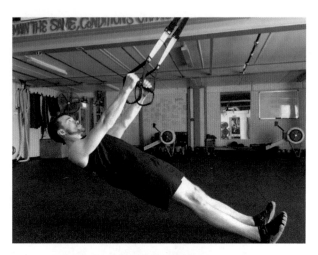

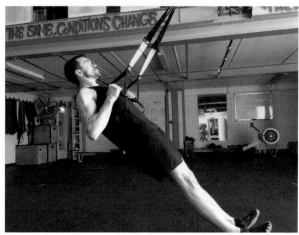

2. Jack-knife Pull-ups 2x20

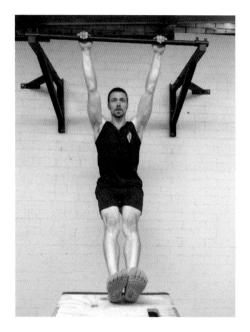

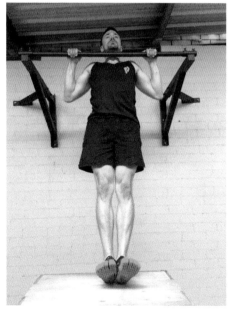

3. Half Pull-ups 2x10

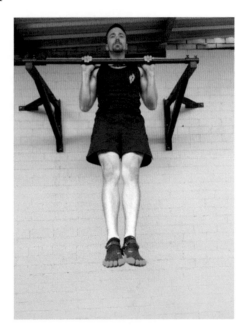

Begin from the top and work your way down to a point where you can comfortably pull yourself back up. Increase the distance to progress to full pull-ups.

4. Full Pull-ups 2x10

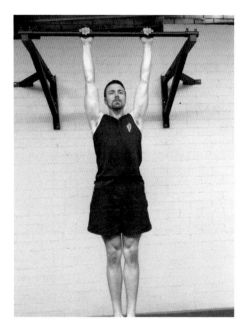

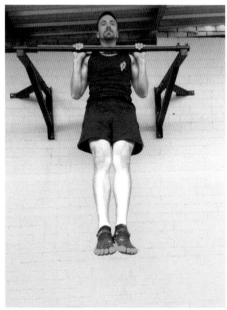

5. Close Pull-ups 2x10

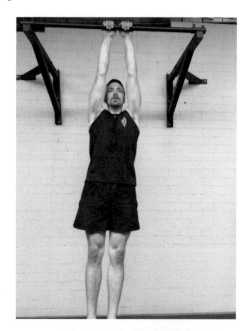

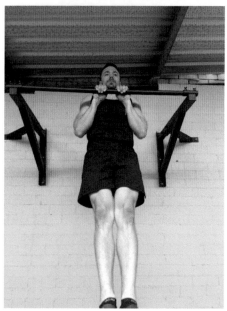

6.   Wrist Hold Pull-ups 2x8

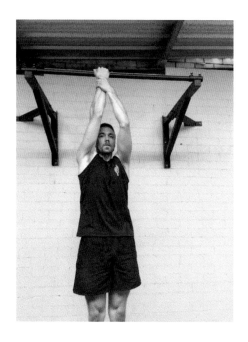

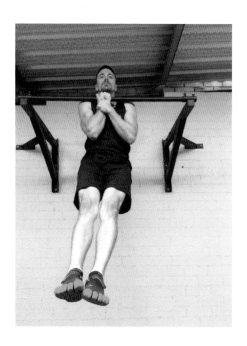

7. Assisted One-Arm Pull-ups 2x4

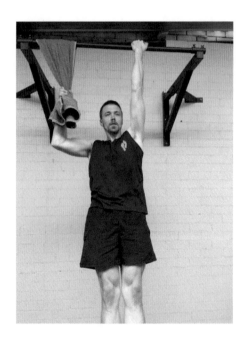

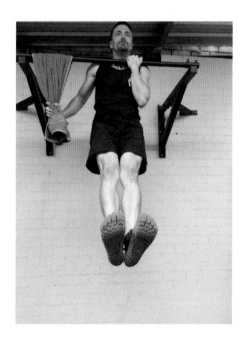

8. One-Arm Pull-up

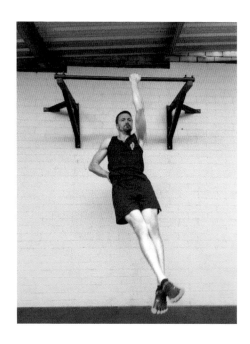

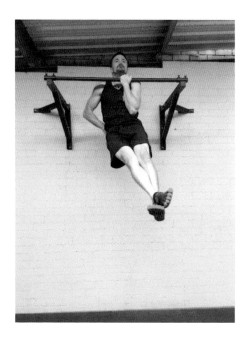

Hanging Leg Raise

1. Bent Leg Raises 2x30

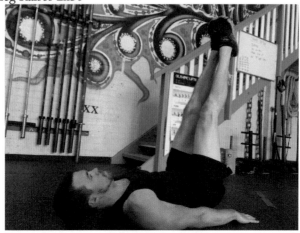

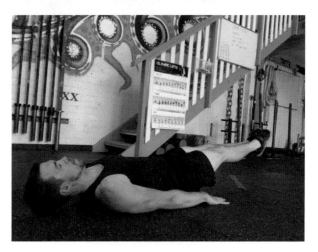

2. Back Body Line Drill 2x10

See Chapter 4 – Bullet Proofing.

3. Hanging Knee Raises 2x10

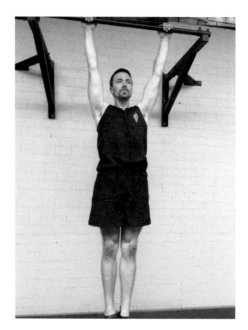

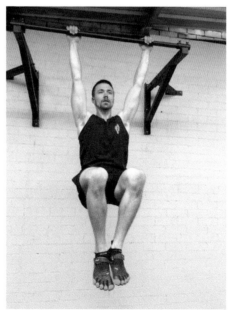

4. Hanging Bent Leg Raises 2x5

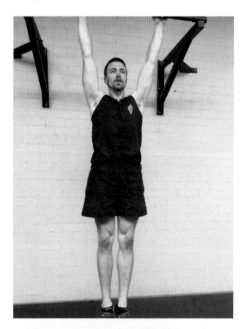

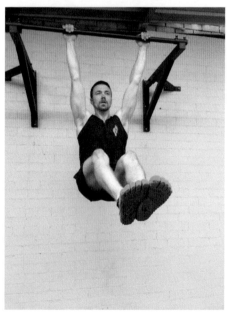

5. Hanging Leg Raise

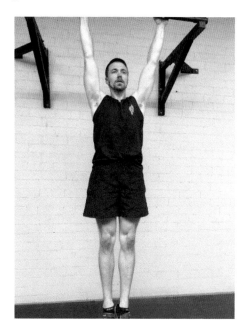

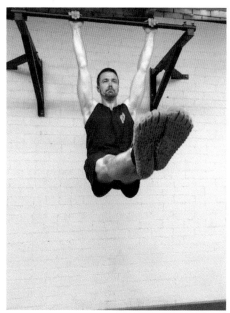

Handstand Push-ups

1. Head Stands 2x1min

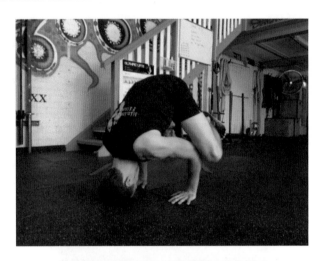

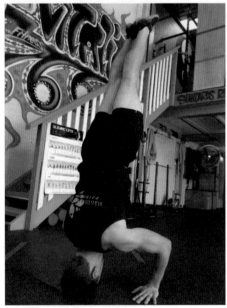

2. Crow stands 2x1min

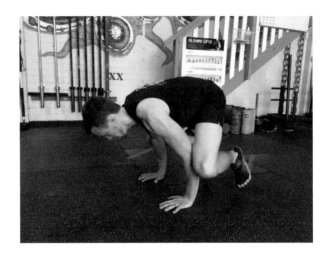

3. Wall Handstand Holds 3x30sec

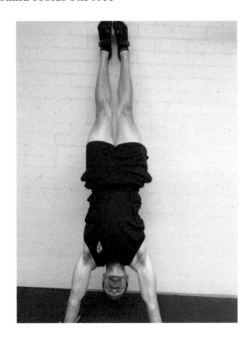

4. Half Handstand Push-ups 2x5

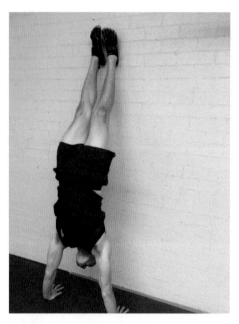

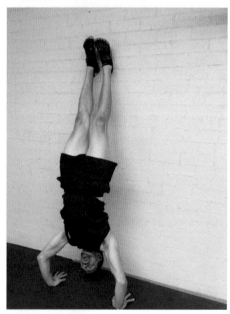

5. Handstand Push-up

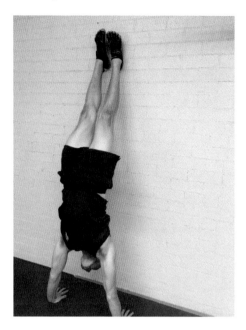

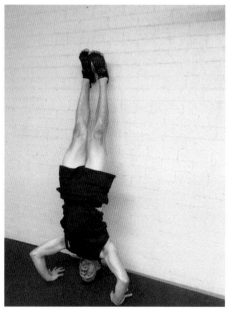

Brett Turley

Bridging

1. Hip Bridge 2x30

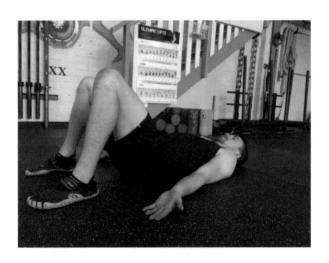

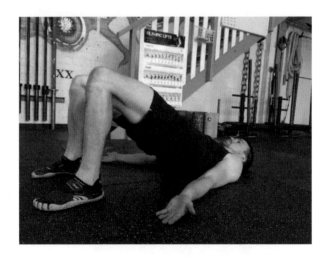

2. Straight Bridge 2x20

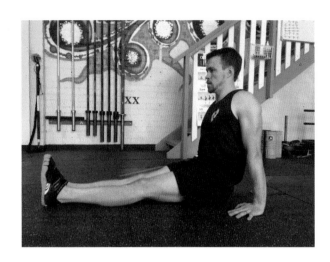

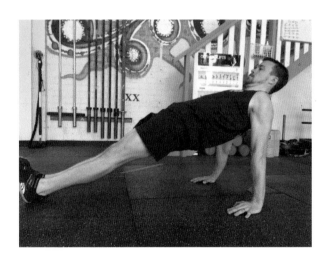

3. Bench Bridge 2x10

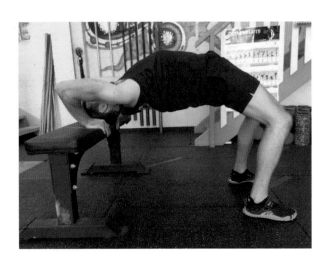

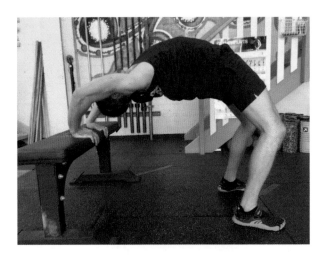

4. Head Bridge 2x10

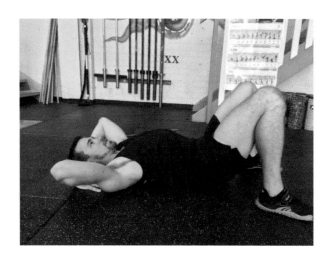

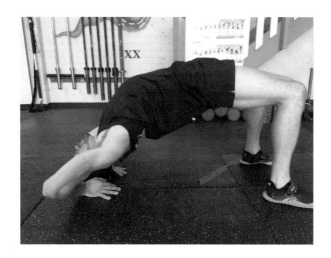

5. Full Bridge

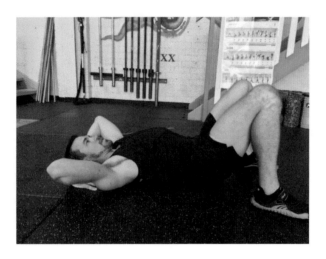

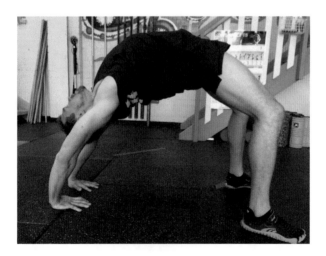

Once you have achieved the last step in the progression sequence you can go a couple of ways. You can add more reps or advance your exercises as far as you want. Recycle the four-week block as many times as you need to achieve the progressions, if you feel like you are stagnating, visit the breaking plateaus section of this book. Strength is a marathon, not a sprint. A great read to push your boundaries and learn great technique would be Paul "Coach" Wade's *Convict Conditioning.*

Jump/Running Progression Plan

Week 1	Week 2	Week 3	Week 4
10 x Broad Jumps	10 x OH Med Ball Toss	10 x Depth Jumps	10 x Depth Jump with Med Ball Throw
3 x 30sec Jump Lunges	3 x 30sec Lateral Jumps (skaters)	5 x Box Jumps 5min work up to Max Height on each	2 x 30sec Lateral Jumps
10 x 100m 1:3 work/rest	6 x 400m 1:2 work/rest	2min Hard/3min Recovery x 4	Beep Test

Brett Turley

Consolidation Work

Push-up Progression Plan (Female)

Beginner <5

Week	1	2	3	4
Set 1	1	2	3	4
2	1	2	3	4
3	1	2	3	4
4	2	3	4	5
5	3	4	5	6
6	3	4	5	6
7	2	3	4	5
8	1	2	3	4
9	1	2	3	4
10	1	2	3	4
Total Reps	16	26	36	46
Completed				

Intermediate <10

Week	1	2	3	4
Set 1	5	6	6	7
2	5	6	6	8
3	5	6	7	9
4	6	7	8	10
5	7	8	9	9
6	7	8	8	8
7	6	7	7	7
8	5	6	6	-
9	5	6	6	-
10	5	6	-	-
Total Reps Completed	56	66	62	58

Brett Turley

Advanced +10

Week	1	2	3	4
Set 1	8	9	10	10
2	9	9	10	10
3	10	10	10	10
4	10	10	10	10
5	10	10	10	10
6	9	10	10	10
7	8	9	10	10
8	-	9	10	10
9	-	-	-	10
10	-	-	-	10
Total Reps	64	76	80	100

Completed

Push-up Progression Plan (Male)

Beginner <10

Week	1	2	3	4
Set 1	8	9	10	10
2	9	9	10	10
3	10	10	10	10
4	10	10	10	10
5	10	10	10	10
6	9	10	10	10
7	8	9	10	10
8	-	9	10	10
9	-	-	-	10
10	-	-	-	10
Total Reps Completed	64	76	80	100

Brett Turley

Intermediate <20

Week	1	2	3	4
Set 1	8	10	12	14
2	10	10	14	14
3	10	12	14	16
4	12	12	16	16
5	14	14	16	18
6	14	14	16	18
7	12	12	16	16
8	10	12	14	16
9	10	10	14	14
10	8	10	12	14
Total Reps	108	116	144	156

Completed

Advanced +20

Week	1	2	3	4
Set 1	16	18	20	20
2	16	18	20	20
3	18	20	20	22
4	18	20	20	22
5	20	20	20	24
6	20	20	20	24
7	18	20	20	22
8	18	20	20	22
9	16	18	20	20
10	16	18	20	20
Total Reps	176	192	200	216

Completed

Brett Turley

Pull-up Progression Plan (Female)

Beginner 0

Week	1	2	3	4
Set 1	10sec SH	15sec SH	20sec SH	30sec SH
2	10sec SH	15sec SH	20sec SH	30sec SH
3	10sec SH	15sec SH	20sec SH	30sec SH
4	10sec SH	15sec SH	20sec SH	30sec SH
5	EL	EL	15 IR	5sec EL
6	EL	EL	15 IR	5sec EL
7	EL	15 IR	15 IR	15 IR
8	EL	15 IR	15 IR	15 IR
9	10 IR	15 IR	15 IR	15 IR
10	10 IR	15 IR	15 IR	15 IR
Total Reps Completed	-	-	-	-

SH – Static Hold **EL** – Eccentric Lower **IR** – Inverted Row

Intermediate <3

Week	1	2	3	4
Set 1	1	1	1	1
2	1	2	2	3
3	1	1	2	2
4	1	1	1	1
5	10sec SH	15sec SH	20sec SH	30sec SH
6	10sec SH	15sec SH	20sec SH	30sec SH
7	10sec SH	15sec SH	20sec SH	30sec SH
8	10sec SH	15sec SH	20sec SH	30sec SH
9	15 IR	20 IR	20 IR	20 IR
10	15 IR	20 IR	20 IR	20 IR
Total Reps	4	5	6	7

Completed

Brett Turley

Advanced +3

Week	1	2	3	4
Set 1	1	1	1	1
2	1	1	1	1
3	2	2	1	2
4	2	2	2	2
5	1	2	2	3
6	1	1	2	3
7	-	1	2	2
8	-	-	1	2
9	-	-	1	1
10	-	-	1	1
Total Reps	8	10	14	18

Completed

Pull-up Progression Plan (Male)

Beginner <5

Week	1	2	3	4
Set 1	1	1	1	2
2	1	1	2	2
3	2	2	2	3
4	2	2	3	3
5	2	3	3	4
6	2	3	3	4
7	1	2	3	3
8	1	2	2	3
9	-	1	2	2
10	-	1	1	2
Total Reps	12	18	22	28

Completed

Brett Turley

Intermediate <10

Week	1	2	3	4
Set 1	4	5	6	7
2	4	5	6	7
3	5	6	7	8
4	5	6	7	8
5	6	7	8	9
6	6	7	8	9
7	5	6	7	8
8	5	6	7	8
9	4	5	6	7
10	4	5	6	7
Total Reps	48	58	68	78

Completed

Advanced +10

Week	1	2	3	4
Set 1	8	9	10	12
2	8	9	10	12
3	8	10	12	14
4	8	10	12	14
5	10	12	14	16
6	10	12	14	16
7	8	10	12	14
8	8	10	12	14
9	8	9	10	12
10	8	9	10	12
Total Reps	84	100	116	136

Completed

Brett Turley

Squat Progression Plan (Male & Female)

Beginner <20

Week	1	2	3	4
Set 1	10	12	14	16
2	10	12	14	16
3	12	14	16	18
4	12	14	16	18
5	14	16	18	20
6	14	16	18	20
7	12	14	16	18
8	12	14	16	18
9	10	12	14	16
10	10	12	14	16
Total Reps	116	136	156	176

Completed

Intermediate <40

Week	1	2	3	4
Set 1	16	18	20	22
2	16	18	20	22
3	18	20	22	24
4	18	20	22	24
5	20	22	24	26
6	20	22	24	26
7	18	20	22	24
8	18	20	22	24
9	16	18	20	22
10	16	18	20	22
Total Reps Completed	176	196	216	236

Brett Turley

Advanced +40

Week	1	2	3	4
Set 1	20	22	24	26
2	20	22	24	26
3	22	24	26	28
4	22	24	26	28
5	24	26	28	30
6	24	26	28	30
7	22	24	26	28
8	22	24	26	28
9	20	22	24	26
10	20	22	24	26
Total Reps	216	236	256	276

Completed

7 KETTLEBELL FUNDAMENTALS

Goal: Kettlebell Skills Acquisition

Practice makes perfect. Incorrect, perfect practice makes perfect. For 4 weeks, this program will help you practice the important fundamental 6 moves with your kettlebells. If you do not have a sound ability to use kettlebells refer to rule 5 of points to remember – Get a God Damn Coach. This will accelerate your learning and skill acquisition and will save you injury down the track, look at it as an investment in your health. The skills that you will practice in the 4 weeks are:

- **The Swing,**
- **The Get Up,**
- **The Clean,**
- **The Press,**
- **The Squat and;**
- **The Snatch.**
-

You are to break it down into weeklong blocks, you are not allowed to fail at a rep or push into anything above your 70-80% effort. You are to "Grease The Groove" or GTG. This training methodology can be found in Pavel Tsatsouline's amazing book *The Naked Warrior* where he focuses on two moves only, the bodyweight pistol and the one arm push-up. You can also read up on your technique by reading *Enter the Kettlebell* also by Pavel. Your breakdown will look like this:

Brett Turley

Week 1 – Two Handed Swing, Goblet Squat & Get Up

Week 2 – Single Arm Swing & Clean

Week 3 – Clean, Press & Rack Squat

Week 4 – Snatch + revision of all other skills

I cannot stress this enough, once you have been coached you are to **PRACTICE** these for 4 weeks. No "working out" or "going hard" just good old practice. The amount of days in your week you dedicate this is up to you, but if you are practicing and not working out you should be able to perform 4-5 days out of your allocated skills easily. If you feel sore, have a rest day. Ensure you conduct an adequate warm-up before you even partake in your practice for the day.

You are probably looking at this simple breakdown of a four-week program and saying, "you're kidding me right?" but trust me when I say the devil is in the details. Take your time to master these skills and during the later programs your body will thank you for it.

8 KETTLEBELL HELL

Goal: Strength & Conditioning

This is a program I run with my clients only 2-3 times per year. I partner this with a nutrition program that quite often has a massive impact on the participant's life. From here we will just focus on the training but if you would like to a copy of the nutrition guidelines please visit my website. The theory behind the training for Kettlebell Hell is divided over 4 weeks, each targeting a different focus. This program has been inspired by some of the best strength, kettlebell and movement coaches of our time. People like Dan John & Pavel Tsatsouline. This program is so simple, it's that effective you won't believe it until you finish the 30 days; stick to it and you will avoid burnout and over training. The break down looks like this:

Week 1 - Movement (Medium Volume/Low Intensity)

Week 2 - Strength Endurance (High Volume)

Week 3 - Strength (High Intensity)

Week 4 - Performance (High Volume/High Intensity)

Week 5 - Testing & Graduation Workout

Week 5 is a two-day week to assess your improvement over the training period.

Brett Turley

The split of days is up to you but traditionally KBH has been started on a Friday to finish on a Saturday, this seems to be a popular option you can split your 4 days up in any fashion, and these splits work well:

Split 1: Mon, Wed, Fri & Sat

Split 2: Mon, Tues, Thurs & Sat

The program was initially designed off split one, but split two will also work. You must maintain the same split over the whole period.

By now you should have been adequately coached and up skilled yourself through the Kettlebell Fundamentals. There is still time dedicated each day towards skill work, so feel free to "Grease the Groove" before training.

One of the biggest complaints from clients using kettlebells during this program is that they start to tear calluses off their hands. Proper maintenance of your hands throughout the 30 days will be essential for success. File down your calluses so they are smooth and not irritated, a nail file works well but a bunyan file (for your feet) works best.

If you are completing this program to target fat loss with the aid of the nutrition guidelines you should follow these tips when deciding the best time to train but this is a personal preference. Both afternoon and morning have their benefits. If training in the morning, either fast or only eat a small amount of food and that will help in the aid of fat loss. Training in the afternoon will aid in increasing strength because you have fuelled yourself all day. Both effects will take place because of your nutrition plan so do not worry about it too much. Place training in your routine when you know you will be able to do it. Be prepared.

During the training you will notice a percentage value placed against an exercise. This is to tell you how hard you are to train at this particular section. Waving loads throughout your week will ensure long term, maintainable results and will help you avoid over training. The values listed on the training and their meaning:

60% - This is an easy session on the particular exercise. By all means use a heavy weight or challenge yourself but 40% of your time, you should be resting. You are not to fail a single repetition or exercise when at 60%. Take it easy and save it up for another day. Remember, it's putting money in the bank team.

80% - This is where most of your gains and improvements will occur, your bread and butter training if you will. This isn't training to failure, you **must** make every rep but emphasis is on reducing your rest between work sets, increasing the weight or increasing the reps depending on your goals.

100% - This should be pretty self-explanatory. This is where you test yourself. You will only hit this point once a week in a chosen exercise and more often than not they are coupled with a 60% effort on a different exercise. Focus in the session is placed upon this 100% exercise.

Now we apply the rule of common sense. If you are sore or believe an injury may result during a particular session you are to do one or all of the following:

- Reduce the intensity level,
- Regress to an easier exercise,
- Reduce the weight that you are using,
- Increase the rest between exercises,
- Take another day off.

Remember rule 3, of points to remember, don't overdraw your bank account.

A full warm-up and cool down should be administered every session. This is not optional. Your warm-up should include foam rolling/trigger point, movement based warm-up and specific mobility work targeting your session for the day. This can include your skill work.

Cooling down should include foam rolling/trigger point and static stretching. Remember, recovery and good nutrition is more important than the session itself.

Brett Turley

The Break Down:

Week 1 – Movement

Different to the Program Minimum as we are completing four days of training featuring the swing and the get up except day one. Targeting the hip hinge pattern and get up technique. If you need time to work on your hip hinge pattern, switch to two-handed swings. Ideally at the end of this week, your hip hinge pattern should be quite solid and your get up technique should be coming along. You are to rest and use the allocated intensity percentage per day, your 60% day should be the easiest rolling up to as many sets of 10/10 (L/R) single arm swings in ten minutes for the 100% day. The kettlebell can touch the ground between sets.

Day 1

10min – As many sets as possible

10/10 Swings @ 60%

Day 2

10min

5/5 Get Up @ 80%

10min

10/10 Swings @ 80%

Day 3

10min

5/5 Get Up @ 60%

10min

10/10 Swings @ 100%

Day 4

10min

5/5 Get Up @ 100%

10min

10/10 Swings @ 60%

Week 2 – Strength Endurance

This week is all about volume, modeled off Dan John's 10,000 swing workout. Drilling your two handed swings until they are solid and working a strength component within three of the four sessions. You will accumulate 500 swings per session totaling 2000 for the week. Females should be aiming to use a 16kg kettlebell and males should shoot for the 24kg. The strength exercises should be done with single or double kettlebells.

Day 1	Day 2 – Swings only
10 Swings	**10 Swings**
3 Squat	Rest 30 seconds
Rest 30 seconds	**15 Swings**
15 Swings	Rest 30 seconds
2 Squat	**25 Swings**
Rest 30 seconds	Rest 30 seconds
25 Swings	**50 Swings**
1 Squat	Rest 2-3 minutes
Rest 30 seconds	5 times through = 500 Swings
50 Swings	
Rest 2-3 minutes	
5 times through = 500 Swings	

Day 3

10 Swings

3 Press

Rest 30 seconds

15 Swings

2 Press

Rest 30 seconds

25 Swings

1 Press

Rest 30 seconds

50 Swings

Rest 2-3 minutes

5 times through = 500 Swings

Day 4

10 Swings

3 Pull-ups

Rest 30 seconds

15 Swings

2 Pull-ups

Rest 30 seconds

25 Swings

1 Pull-up

Rest 30 seconds

50 Swings

Rest 2-3 minutes

5 times through = 500 Swings

Week 3 – Strength

Armor Building. Reps and formats can be changed but the theory remains the same cleans, presses & squats. Week 3 is a focus on muscular hypertrophy and strength. The aim for the week is to use the heaviest kettlebells possible that you can clean twice, press once and squat three times for multiple sets within the given time frame. The kettlebells can be placed down during the period but emphasis should be placed on equaling or beating the previous days results. Days two and four, consider a reduced time but a weight increase, this is only if you are ready to progress.

Day 1

15min AMRAP (As Many Rounds As Possible)

2 Clean

1 Press

3 Squat

Day 2

10min AMRAP

2 Clean

1 Press

3 Squat

Increase weight

Day 3

20min AMRAP

2 Clean

1 Press

3 Squat

Day 4

15min AMRAP

2 Clean

1 Press

3 Squat

Increase weight

Brett Turley

Week 4 – Performance

This week uses a modified version of Pavel's Rite of Passage. Presses are featured everyday with the volume increasing by ladders over the week. There are also partnered strength elements being the squat and the pull-up. These are done as supersets combining the presses and pull-ups/squats back to back before moving up to another rung.

The swing and snatch serial at the end of the session has a percentage value attached and you are to work to that intensity. If you are not confident with your snatch regress to single or two-handed swings. Weights for the snatch are to be one size lower than your single arm swing kettlebell.

Day 1	Day 2
Press & Pull-up	**Press & Squat**
3x1, 2, 3, 4, 5	**4x1, 2, 3, 4, 5**
5 min*	**5 min***
Snatch/Swing @ 60%	**Swing @** 80%
Day 3	Day 4
Press & Pull-up	**Press & Squat**
4x1, 2, 3, 4, 5	**5x1, 2, 3, 4, 5**
5 min*	**5 min***
Snatch/Swing @ 100%	**Swing @** 60%

*min = minutes

Week 5 Day 1 – Strength Testing

The final week will see only two days of training. Day 1 will be a strength test looking at your 1RM for your kettlebell strength lifts or grinds. You are to work up to a comfortable 1RM for:

Get Up

KB Squat (Double in the rack position)

KB Press (Single Arm)

You should finish this session feeling like you have something left in the tank. Save yourself for the graduation workout.

Day 2 – The Graduation Workout

Our final session for Kettlebell Hell will test everything you have worked on in the last 30 days. You are not to miss a rep on the Get Ups and you are to beat your best amount of rounds for your armor-building ladder from week 3. In relation to the snatch test, if you are still not confident with your technique drop to heavy single arm swings in the same time frame.

5/5 Get Up in 10 Minutes

10 minutes Armor Building Ladder

5 Minute Snatch Test

You are to have 5 minutes rest between all sections during your graduation workout. Make sure you take a couple of days off after the 30-day period has finished, you will need it.

9 MINIMALISTIC RITE OF PASSAGE

Goal: Kettlebell Strength & Skills

This program is probably one of my favorites. It has been modified for one thing, to reduce wear and tear on the shoulders. The old adage is to press lots, you must press lots. I think this isn't quite right for all situations; the volume in the original Rite Of Passage by Pavel is a rather large dose to the old shoulders. In no shadow of a doubt this has worked for hundreds if not thousands of people before me but what if you had previous injuries or limitations like myself that prevented you from being able to complete such high volume pressing? Due to my injury history, I needed a way to achieve a half-bodyweight press without revisiting the hospital or surgery for my shoulder, because that would not be a good choice. From this program I discovered:

To press lots, you must press enough, but find exercises and alternatives that assist your pressing without compromising shoulder health and strength or push you towards injury.

In this case you are still pressing lots but you are missing the massive amount of single arm kettlebell pressing that the original program dictated. You are also working on exercises that promote good shoulder health and there is enough room to adjust when you hit a stage of burnout or come close to injury. The program is broken down into six-week phases, with the built in alternatives to single arm pressing and scheduled deload or taper week in week 5 ensures you can maintain this program for a reasonable duration. The first phase I ever ran of this program, I increased my kettlebell press 40% in two phases. That's 8kg in 12 weeks, from 20kg to

28kg. As my friends know my shoulder history, and being of a small frame (65kg ringing wet), this was a significant jump. It didn't take me long to hit double bodyweight the next time I did this program.

Week 1 – 4: As per program

Week 5: Deload, drop down one size from the current kettlebells you are using for press, swing and snatch and reduce all pressing ladders from 5 to 3.

Week 6: If you are feeling good choose to test yourself on two of the exercises such as the press and the snatch, with the snatch being tested on day 5 of week 6. Let the other exercises progress easily and test a following six weeks later.

Repeat the six-week sequence until you can:

- **Press half your bodyweight**
- **100 reps in 5 min* snatch test 12/16kg for women & 20/24kg for men**
- **Pull-up with 16kg women/24kg men**
- **Show good technique on Windmill, Pistol Squat & Push Press**

*min = minutes

You will be running a five-day training week the best block I have seen work is:

Monday, Tuesday, Wednesday, Thursday & Saturday

Day 1 – Double Kettlebell Press:

Clean & Press Ladder (Double Kettlebells)

5x1, 2, 3

Superset with;

Weighted Pull-ups 9x1 (one for every rung of the ladder)

KB Snatch 5min* @ 50-60%

Brett Turley

Day 2 – Skills Day:

Get Up 5/5 No Time Limit – work to a comfortable 70-80%

Windmill 5x5/5 – Easy weight.

Day 3 – Heavy Single Arm Press:

Clean & Press 5x1/1(L/R)

Superset with;

BW Pull-ups 5x5

Swings 10min* @ 70-80%

Two sizes heavier than snatch size kettlebell

Day 4 – Skills Day:

Pistol – Follow progressions from Evolution of Man

Push press 5min* @70-80%

Day 5 – Single Arm Pressing Volume:

Clean & Press Ladder

5x1, 2, 3, 4, 5

Swings 10min* @ 80-90%

One size heavier than snatch size kettlebell

*min = minutes

During your warm ups, focus on a lot of exercise specific correctives. As there is a lot of shoulder work during the program ensure you have an adequate amount of correctives and exercises that suit your situation. Exercises that work well within your warm-up framework specific to shoulders are:

- Halos,
- Arm Bars,
- Scapular Setting Drills,
- Handstand holds, handstand push-ups and,
- Bottom's up kettlebell presses, carries and squats.

Don't forget your other work, preparation for your swings, snatches and pistols will all be necessary throughout your program. As stated in the correctives section, you can substitute your rest with corrective work to help get an adequate amount in your training session.

10 MINIMALIST BARBELL CYCLE

Goal: Build Strength

The target of this barbell program is simple. To get strong. This is where you will reach most of the standards mentioned when it comes to strength if you haven't hit them already. The idea is simple, use the big three lifts, squat, bench and deadlift as your main lift or work for the three-day per week program and use the supplement exercises to help keep your body in good order and assist you along the way.

The big three will be utilizing a few principles from Dan John's *Easy Strength*.

The Rule of 10 – Conduct no more than ten work repetitions of the big three on the given days. To keep things varied enough to ensure progress you will change your sets and reps every week over the six week period:

Week 1 – 3x3

Week 2 – 2x5

Week 3 – 5-3-2

Week 4 – 5x2

Week 5 – 6x1

Week 6 – 5x2 (Easy 70%)

5 Minutes rest between work sets – You are to have 5 minutes rest between your working sets of the big three. Strength is a practice, not a race.

Work between 80-90% 1RM – During your work sets you are to stick in between 80-90% of your 1RM. You may notice that there is no "testing" week in your program. Only test once in a blue moon, other than that when the weight feels easy, you move up. Always leave a rep or two in the bank. If you do test for a PB, have two weeks of easy training following the lift.

Finish stronger than what you started – This will be what you use to gauge how hard to push. If you feel strong stick to the plan, if you feel flat don't be afraid to back it off a bit and save it for another day.

Assistance work is just that, assistance – Use the assistance work on the days given as easy strength following your big three. Do not ignore these lifts or movements but work at an easy 70% capacity.

Day 1

Front Squat - Rule of 10

Pull-ups - 5x5

Get Ups - 3/3

Ab-wheel Rollouts - 2x5

Day 2

Bench Press - Rule of 10

Renegade Lunge - 5x3/3

Hanging Leg Raise - 2x5

Swings - 1x50

Brett Turley

Day 3

Deadlift - Rule of 10

KB Shoulder Press - 5x5

Bat Wing Rows - 3x5

Asymmetrical Loaded Carry 4x30-50m

As you can see during a week you will cover push, pull, hip hinge, squat, loaded carry and everything else such as straight arm strength and corrective work at least a couple of times. It is a well-balanced approach to general strength. On the second six week phase of the program I want you to switch your big three exercises. Switch them to:

Front Squat to Back Squat,

Bench Press to Barbell Shoulder Press and,

Deadlift to Romanian Deadlift.

This may seem a bit odd but switching exercises after six weeks will have you training same but different. You will be able to work harder on the squat while the deadlift takes a break. This has seen the longevity of clients improve as when they plateau, they change just enough to push through. The press also has a great cross over for athletic endeavors, switch your kettlebell press on day 3 to kettlebell or barbell floor press in your second six week cycle.

The asymmetrical loaded carry can be done one of three ways, suitcase, rack or waiters/overhead. You can vary these from week to week as you see fit but you are already working straight-arm strength overhead using the get up and hanging leg raise in your program. The suitcase or farmers would be my pick to work.

In season athletes – Reduce the volume of your reps by one third but keep the intensity (weight) the same. This will change your Rule of 10 to Rule of 6. Rep schemes will look like 3x2, 2x3 3-2-1 and so on. You are also to drop back to two days a week meaning you will cycle through like this:

Week 1: Day 1 & Day 2

Week 2: Day 3 & Day 1

Week 3 Day 2 & Day 3

When training during a season, don't be afraid to back the big three off occasionally if you are starting to push near fatigue or injury or needing the extra energy for your sport. If your pre-season preparation has been sufficient, you shouldn't have a problem. You will be able to dedicate more time and energy into your sports specific skills. A great way to ensure you are pushing the boundaries mid season is to re-adjust your 1RM like this:

Your in season 1 RM is 90% of your off season 1RM or 100%. For example:

Your true 1RM is 160kg

Your mid season 1RM becomes 144kg @ 90%

Your working weight at 80% is now 115kg

To avoid burnout even further, substitute this program with a 2 week Prehab block every now and then. It will give you time to let aches and pains settle down and for you to focus more on the sport or skill at hand.

The Renegade Lunge

Day two of the barbell cycle sees an interesting exercise being the Renegade Lunge. I got this beauty out of Pavel's *Beyond Bodybuilding* and it is hands down one of the best lateral strength developers that I have used. The idea is simple, set up a bar at chest height on a power rack or similar set up. You are then to stand side onto the bar holding either one or two kettlebells. You are then to step under and across to the other side of the bar returning to the standing position. Do not get pulled down or forward you are stepping to the side on which the bar is situated. This is a great exercise for any athlete that needs lateral speed, strength or movement in their chosen sport.

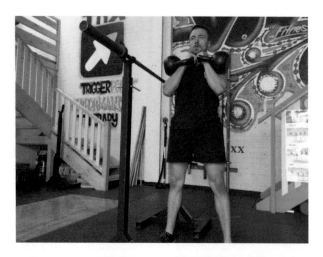

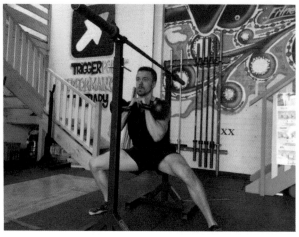

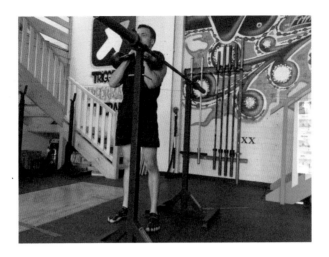

11 MINIMALISTIC TIPS & TECHNIQUES

Tips For A Bigger Kettlebell Press

It's not just about muscle or brute strength, moving up that ladder in kettlebell sizes for pressing requires, patience and mastery of technique. Now I will say that some people are just pressing freaks but if you are anything like me, pressing a heavy bell such as half bodyweight requires more than just screaming and hope. Here is the pressing checklist:

For The Clean:
- Firm grip (do not re-grip for the entire press)
- Drive with Glutes

In The Rack:
- Hips under/Glutes on
- Feet move in closer/Stomp
- Shoulders engaged (Down and back)

For The Press:
- Glutes on/Knees locked
- Firm Grip
- Eyes on KB
- Compress Chest
- Force forearm against KB
- Don't stop - Hiss through teeth to push through sticking points
- Trigger/Squeeze with your spare hand through sticking points
- Don't exaggerate "J" pattern
- Push yourself away from the bell

Always Start Bad Side First

When conducting any unilateral or asymmetrical exercises, start your bad side first. This will let you be as fresh as possible to focus on technique and it will let you finish strong on your good side. Most people will have a preferred or better side when it comes to asymmetrical lifting.

Breaking plateaus

Tip 1: Take A Rest Or Have an Easy Day/s.

If you are struggling with the volume during your training or believe that you are getting close to injury or burn out choose to either rest or take an easy day. A rest day doesn't necessarily mean having it off but try working your correctives and having a light session. An easy day means dropping the reps, load or increasing the rest period. We also call this a deload session or week. Don't be afraid to work at only 50% capacity. Enjoy the movement.

Tip 2: Consolidation Training

Consolidation training refers to increasing your working sets. Still apply the adequate warm up but increase your work sets accordingly. This does NOT mean going all out. Increasing your work sets by one or two will help your body break past your sticking point in training. It goes without saying but do not do this if you are on the way to burn out or injury.

Strength Is A Practice

Strength isn't a race; everyone will adapt and advance differently. Do not compare yourself to others when you are training. Take your time to master technique before intensity, you will surpass all the others that race ahead of you or skip the crucial initial steps by remaining injury free and therefore being able to train in the long run.

Don't Be Afraid To Move On

When you are working your way through this book and the program, if you are starting to burn out on a particular program do not be afraid to finish the cycle you are on and move to another phase of training. Phases of training in this book last between 4-6 weeks. The reason for this is that the body will cease to adapt to stimulus after about six weeks. You have not failed a program if you do not hit the standards in the first phase. If you have improved from where you started during your phase this deems it successful. There is nothing wrong with moving to a different focus within the book to give your body time to wind down and practice something else. Your longevity within training will increase and you will enjoy yourself more by doing this, we don't want to be flogging our heads against a brick wall. Like I said, strength is a practice and not a race. Take your time and don't be afraid to move on and then revisit a program down the track. A lot of my clients practice this and find they improve on certain skills without even training for them. A well-rounded, structured program will have this effect or at least keep your body in relatively good shape.

Loading Waves

Ensure adequate preparation is made to load your waves between your workouts, training weeks and programs. You will not be able to maintain an intense rate for very long. Set your standards at:

50-60% - Easy day/week. Enjoy going through your warm-up and session leaving plenty in the tank. You should leave feeling like you haven't done enough. This is the sort of day you implement to avoid injury or burnout or before testing.

70-80% - Bread and Butter. This is where most of your gains in training will occur. You can afford to have a majority of these during your week or program. Be sure to back it off when necessary. You should leave your session feeling stronger than what you came in. You can even get a bit of a sweat up.

90%+ - The Proving Grounds. This is where you put all you have been practicing together to find new 1RM or performance levels. If you are working this into your program, only have one 90% session/week until you can afford to push. Leave your 100% for game day or testing once every 3 months or so.

When to go all out?

Rarely ever. Save this stuff for the times it really counts. Being in the gym grunting and screaming every session doesn't help progress and also makes you look like a tool. Save your stuff for the big game or when it really counts. No one will ever remember the guy who PB'd in training but blew his game or competition out of his arse when it counted. Dan John states it beautifully in *Intervention*:

"Strive for a quiet head, efficient movements and a sense of calm when training."

Opposites Attract In Assistance Exercises

When training and you want to add supersets or assistance exercises in strength or conditioning environment choose exercises that complement the main lift or each other. For instance, if you are deadlifting, choose an exercise like goblet squats as they can be used as a corrective or assistance exercise. As for where to add power development exercises, you might need to buy my next book.

Eat Like an Adult

A note on nutrition, a lot of great coaches say this, and a lot of people profess to have this philosophy, we are 100% right. Eat like a god damn adult. You don't need fancy meal plans or diets. Whole foods such as vegetables, meat and a little bit of fruit will go a long way. Add some healthy fats and plenty of water into the mix and you are on the money. Hell, you could even add some grains in there and you won't die. Stop your complaining about being overweight and get it done. 99% of people have no excuse as to why they are overweight except for being lazy or stupid. Or both. For those that have actual illnesses like metabolic disorders and thyroid conditions, educate yourself as best you can for your particular situation. My wife has Hashimotos Disease, which means her body is eating her thyroid; she will not have one in the future. And she isn't overweight, because she eats like an adult. If this statement offends you, ask yourself these questions:

Have I educated myself enough towards my situation?

Have I done enough to improve my situation?

If you answer no to either or both of these, get off your behind and start improving your own situation. Nobody but you can make the difference.

Brett Turley

FURTHER READING & EDUCATION

For bodyweight skills & breathing technique;
The Naked Warrior – Pavel
Convict Conditioning – Paul Wade

For the kettlebell enthusiasts;
Enter The Kettlebell – Pavel
Simple & Sinister – Pavel

For Strength & Athletic performance:
Beyond Bodybuilding – Pavel
Easy Strength – Dan John & Pavel

For the trainer:
Intervention – Dan John

For movement:
Movement – Gray Cook & Lee Burton

Courses Worth Attending:
Russian Kettlebell Certification (RKC)
Strong First Certification (SFG)
Functional Movement Screen Level 1 & 2
Anything that sparks your interest and anything with above mentioned
authors and coaches.

"You should always be adding tools to your tool box."

ABOUT THE AUTHOR

His friends and family call him professional, committed and reliable, to his face anyway. He is an avid coffee drinker, dog lover and is rather fond of his wife, when she's not angry… His minimalistic approach to health & fitness, love of sarcasm and a disdain for stupidity has transformed countless clients into the people they want to be by doing less. Specializing in Kettlebells, Rehab and Functional Movement he really believes that Less is More. And he can prove it.

From being blown up inside an armored vehicle, being shot at and looking for bombs in Afghanistan to dislocating shoulders before debut boxing bouts. Mr. Minimalism has done it all, well the stupid stuff anyway. Now he enjoys being able to move pain free and move a heap of weight generally in the form of a kettlebell, when he feels the need. He also likes teaching people how to do the same.

Printed in Great Britain
by Amazon.co.uk, Ltd.,
Marston Gate.